KU-624-215

Risk Assessment and Management for Living Well with Dementia

Charlotte L. Clarke, Heather Wilkinson,
John Keady and Catherine E. Gibb

Foreword by Professor Murna Downs

Jessica Kingsley *Publishers*
London and Philadelphia

Contains public sector information licensed under the Open Government Licence v1.0.
Table 2.1 from Clarke and Heyman 1998 on p.26 is adapted by permission of Hodder and Stoughton
Limited/Edward Arnold (Publishers) Limited/Hodder Education.
Table 4.1 from Manthorpe and Moriarty 2010 on p.89 is adapted by permission of Jill Manthorpe.
Figure 4.1 from Manthorpe and Moriarty 2010 on p.90 is reproduced by permission of Jill Manthorpe.
Figure 5.2 from Clarke and Gardner 2002 on p.102 is reproduced by permission of Hawker
Publications.

First published in 2011
by Jessica Kingsley Publishers
116 Pentonville Road
London N1 9JB, UK
and
400 Market Street, Suite 400
Philadelphia, PA 19106, USA

www.jkp.com

Copyright © Charlotte L. Clarke, Heather Wilkinson, John Keady and Catherine E. Gibb 2011
Foreword copyright © Murna Downs 2011
Printed digitally since 2013

All rights reserved. No part of this publication may be reproduced in any material form (including
photocopying or storing it in any medium by electronic means and whether or not transiently
or incidentally to some other use of this publication) without the written permission of the
copyright owner except in accordance with the provisions of the Copyright, Designs and Patents
Act 1988 or under the terms of a licence issued by the Copyright Licensing Agency Ltd, Saffron
House, 6–10 Kirby Street, London EC1N 8TS. Applications for the copyright owner's written
permission to reproduce any part of this publication should be addressed to the publisher.

Warning: The doing of an unauthorised act in relation to a copyright work
may result in both a civil claim for damages and criminal prosecution.

Library of Congress Cataloging in Publication Data
Risk assessment and management for living well with dementia / Charlotte L. Clarke ... [et al.].
    p. cm.
Includes bibliographical references and index.
ISBN 978-1-84905-005-0 (alk. paper)
1. Dementia--Patients--Care. 2. Decision making. 3. Risk
management. I. Clarke, Charlotte L. (Charlotte Laura)
RC521.R49 2011
616.8'3--dc22
                            2010044477

British Library Cataloguing in Publication Data
A CIP catalogue record for this book is available from the British Library

ISBN 978 1 84905 005 0
eISBN 978 0 85700 519 9

Contents

PART III RISK AND YOUR PRACTICE

Foreword

Risk Assessment and Management for Living Well with Dementia could not be more timely. Living well with dementia is now a priority for the Department of Health in England as indeed it is throughout most of the world. Living well for all of us requires that we identify and negotiate risks in our lives. As such, risk management is central to wellbeing and quality of life. We are encouraged to think of risk not as something to be avoided and from which we need to shy away, but rather as something integral to wellbeing which needs to be embraced and actively managed. Risk is not an abstract and unitary concept which we wish to remove, but a complex and continually negotiated aspect of all of our lives.

In *Risk Assessment and Management for Living Well with Dementia* we are reminded that risk looks different from different perspectives and that these perspectives in turn are informed by different knowledge bases. While professionals and practitioners may have one view of risk, family members may have another and people with dementia will, in turn, have their own perspective. This guide challenges us to address the complexity of different understandings of, and perspectives on, risk. It provides helpful guidance on how we might reconcile our perspective with other perspectives, most notably those of people with dementia. As such, the authors encourage us to take as our starting point in risk management the perspective and needs of people with dementia. By grounding this contemporary good practice guide in the experience of four people with dementia, *Risk Assessment and Management for Living Well with Dementia* illustrates how we need to ground our concern with risk assessment and management in the context of the person's life – their life history, family circumstance, and social and cultural context.

Risk is not only integral to our personal lives and day-to-day wellbeing but also to professional practice. *Risk Assessment and Management for Living Well with Dementia* discusses dilemmas present in our day-to-day professional practice and offers a basic legislative framework within which to consider our everyday practice. The guide stresses that successful resolution of risk dilemmas in dementia care requires the inclusion of the perspective, needs, rights and entitlements of people with dementia.

Usefully portraying risk assessment and management from two main perspectives – that of people with dementia and their family members, and that of managers and practitioners – the authors provide a risk framework for dementia which focuses on the following four elements:

- identifying the risks in the context of the person's biography and life history

- identifying the risks to the various stakeholders, including professionals, practitioners, family and the person with dementia

- weighing the different risks involved

- identifying current and past strategies for managing risks.

In summary, *Risk Assessment and Management for Living Well with Dementia* raises a range of contemporary issues and concerns which require our attention. It not only raises these issues and concerns, however, but also proposes a clear way forward for person-centred risk assessment and management seeking to reconcile the differing perspectives of practitioners, family members and people with dementia.

Professor Murna Downs
Series Editor of Bradford Dementia Group Good Practice Guides
University of Bradford
14 March 2011

PART I
INTRODUCTION

Chapter 1

Key Issues in Risk and Dementia Care

INTRODUCTION

Risk has multiple meanings for multiple people in multiple situations. When risk is linked to dementia and to services, it is perhaps not surprising that the language can become emotive and a person with dementia start to be defined in terms of their 'risk behaviour', the 'levels of risk they pose' or the outcomes of their 'risk assessment'. In so many ways, minimising risk and maximising 'safe' practice are fast becoming watchwords of 'successful' dementia care practice. As an illustration, one person living with young onset dementia, who was speaking at one of our risk project awareness events, shared a story about statutory services stopping a day care activity of swimming at the local swimming pool as their risk assessment had revealed that his safety in the water 'could no longer be guaranteed'. However, as a citizen and local taxpayer, he would often enter the (same) local swimming pool, pay an admission fee, get changed, put his clothes in one of those lockers that never quite works, and swim. Afterwards, he would then get dry, change, meet his wife and have a coffee in the café area of the swimming pool. He had no shame in informing the attendants he had dementia. The pool attendants then supported his swimming activity and would help him locate his locker should matching the number on the wristband to the number on the locker prove to be a problem. It was all done openly and supportively. However, for services, somehow the process between responding to a request for a 'normal' activity and then calculating the level of risk it posed became distorted with the result that the younger person with dementia was no longer in charge of a decision that impacted upon his daily life and, perhaps more important, his quality of life.

Life stories, meanings and autonomy come together to create points at which services make critical decisions. Life is about making judgements and decisions that impact on our lives and those closest to us. For people living with dementia, those judgements and decisions, as the swimming pool example illustrates, move from a private, internal dialogue about 'what is best for me' to an open public/professional debate about 'what is best for him'. Other people have an opinion, a duty and responsibility for the 'risk'. This opening chapter rehearses the causes and consequences of these debates and examines the notion of risk as it is lived day by day by people with dementia, their close family members and their community networks.

LIVING AND RISK

We all have a notion of what our life is and how we want it to be lived. Life is filled with our hopes and our relationships, our expectations and our responsibilities. It is something familiar to us and has a certain rhythm and routine – a form and purpose which recurs every day. This form and purpose of day-to-day life differs for us all, sometimes to such an extent that we may think of other people's lives as being quite strange and not at all like our own. But there is always a form and purpose – one we set out, by and large, to replicate day after day throughout our lives.

Our everyday life is also the stage on which the trials, tribulations and joys of our lives take place. Most often this is shared through the other people in our lives – very often it is caused by the other people in our lives. It is as a result of these relationships that our everyday life shapes and reshapes over time, causing happiness, tensions or major upheavals. Such events may be the routines of work, family life, shopping, caring and so on. Events may be joyous, such as the birth of a child in the family, or unwanted and forced upon us, such as a bereavement.

Invariably, our response to such events is to accommodate and adapt. However, we are not alone in doing this; others who experience the same events will also seek to accommodate and adapt. As a consequence, we enter a complex arena in which we and others are adapting and, simultaneously, we are all adapting to each other. So, as we take a step to adapt, others may comment, change their position, support and challenge our move, and seek to moderate it. This process, known as *reflexive positioning*, is one key element in understanding risk in dementia care.

There are two aspects to reflexive positioning, which parallel the form and purpose described above. First, the way we conduct our everyday life is shaped by us and by those around us and we adapt it according to the everyday lives of others. Second, the way in which we understand our life and its purpose is shaped by our past and our future as they cast their influence on our present. These two aspects of reflexive positioning lead to what we have called the *contested territories* of everyday life.

Let us explain this more clearly through the life of Jane, who participated in a study we did. Jane is a retired teacher who has had a stroke and who has dementia. She lives with her partner Peter. Their everyday life was made up of Jane wanting to do things she had always done (go to the shops, do the washing up, smoking, and so on) and Peter feeling more and more worried about Jane doing some of these things. As a result, Peter felt that he needed to monitor her activities in order to keep her safe. In response to his vigilance, Jane attempted to do things behind his back. This reflexive positioning meant that, for Jane and Peter, everyday life was becoming something that was an ongoing battleground – a contested territory.

We can use risk theory and ideas to help us understand and explain some of these issues. Two of the main ideas we will explore are *risk perception* and *risk construction* – in other words, how someone identifies, understands and describes the challenges and opportunities that they are faced with and how they then adapt; and moreover, how they do so through reflexive positioning. We will also explore how different people, or stakeholders, will have a different view of risks and one of the key challenges is in identifying these different views, enabling people with dementia to express their view(s) and in making decisions that take these sometimes competing views into account. We will explore how, as practitioners, risk can be assessed with a view to proactive management of the contested territory that is causing concern or dispute.

LIVING WELL WITH DEMENTIA

People who live with dementia may experience family, friends and service providers as framing their situation as 'tragic' and/or 'problematic', with associated risks framed as 'unwanted' and 'undesirable'. However, this assumption of the situation as tragic can be challenged. A counter-narrative (or alternative storyline) has led to the development of person-centred care for people with dementia, and if we are to promote living well with dementia we must ensure that our understanding of risk is based on a person-centred counter-narrative. To explain this a little more, a counter-narrative was found in a study of people with alcohol-related brain damage (Keady *et al.* 2009) where instead of the 'tragic' stories that one would expect to hear, including seemingly adverse and life-threatening events, people living with alcohol-related brain damage shared an expectation of hope and recovery as they had seen other people 'improve' and 'go home'. It is also known that providing home care for a person with dementia can bring families and relationships closer together, which is a counter-narrative to the 'strain and 'burden' that is often talked about in describing the lives of family carers. Similarly, Oulton and Heyman (2009) reported on a study in which parents of disabled children describe the initial shock of learning of their child's disability – but they describe the life-enhancing experience of caring for a disabled child.

Bury's (1991) work in relation to biographical disruption and accommodation is particularly helpful in explaining these processes – the 'catastrophic' event or diagnosis which forces a disruption to someone's past and future life story, and the subsequent reconciliation (or search for meaning) which leads to adjustment, or accommodation, in their biographical narrative. Through thinking of dementia as a biographical disruption in or to someone's life, it may be possible to identify hope, optimism, recovery and enhancement. In dementia care, we are well placed and experienced in working with people's biographies through life story work and such activities can be used to promote and instil hope, a primary element in recovery and living well with the condition, as outlined in the National Dementia Strategy in England (Department of Health 2009).

On the other hand, the catastrophic model of dementia may lead to a resistance from practitioners to engaging with risk and an inability to promote positive risk taking because of the organisational and professional culture which staff and managers practise and perpetuate. The risk-adverse, or safety-first, approach of some service providers may indeed compromise developing more effective services (Titterton 2005). For some, removing physical risk results in also removing components of life that are valued and so compromises quality of life – we can call these compromises *silent harms* because they are so much harder to recognise than a physical event such as falling or getting lost.

Fundamentally, both models of risk – as problematic and as contributing to quality of life – do not deal fully with the contradictions and paradoxes inherent in living with dementia in a disabling society, which has the potential to accelerate the restriction of choice and decision making (Swain, French and Cameron 2003). Neither model takes into account the interplay between self and society, between the potential difficulties accompanying living with dementia and the context in which it takes place.

A further way in which risk can be a double-edged sword in relation to quality of life concerns the ways in which risk is used to promote safety but is also, and in contradiction, used to promote autonomy. The perpetual tension between these uses of risk is seen in the work of Fortinsky, Panzer and Wakefield (2009) in which older people may be driven to an 'unrealistic' framing of their risk of falling by a desire to remain independent at home and in control of their environment. It is through such sense-making processes that people rationalise their engagement with (potentially) health-harming activities.

Underpinning this tension is concern about where the responsibility for risk management rests – who assumes or relinquishes responsibility for the balance of protecting safety and promoting autonomy. This responsibility may be ascribed, that is, 'given' to someone or a group by others or by society. For example, Powell, Wahidin and Zinn (2007) identify how risk theory enables an understanding of how older people are rendered 'subjects' of society: 'risk is the intended outcome of a range of social practices whose aim is the management of a population that is useful, productive and self-managing' (p.73).

Despite these moves towards greater responsibility of individuals, as seen in the United Kingdom (UK) personalisation agenda, contemporary health care privileges the knowledge held by health and social care practitioners and underplays the importance of knowledge held by service users. Most disenfranchised by this weighting of knowledge are the general public and those with long-term conditions, particularly those living with dementia, who are prone to be stigmatised as a result (Alzheimer's Society 2008). For people with dementia the presence of such an impairment can undermine their very sense of self. In the research by Keady *et al.* (2009), for example, alcohol-related brain damage was assimilated as a component and projection of self and identity (one participant describing himself as a 'Korsakoff's creep', a reference to his identification as having Korsakoff dementia). Concerns about social exclusion are restricted by the failure of technical-rational health care models to address the complex socio-economic and biographical concerns of people with dementia and their families. There is a failure to recognise the different knowledge bases in managing health and ill-health and the work engaged in by people to contextualise the received knowledge in creating and recreating their sense of self. People are, however, risk experts in their own right and they exercise their expertise through self-management and what services may perceive to be 'non-compliance'.

Risk theory, perception and management are central to concepts of choice and the capacity to execute decisions. A focus on physical safety only is likely to be detrimental to the overall wellbeing of an individual and their family (Clarke *et al.* 2006). It is essential to realise the therapeutic benefit of optimal risk engagement and to recognise that the risk experiences of someone with a long-term condition are shaped by social and cultural forces across the globe – and are fundamentally shaped by the relationship between individuals, institutions and society. This intersects with the emerging public health focus on prevention through promoting resilience in individuals and forms a further aspect of the individualisation of responsibility.

In summary, the ability of someone to live well with dementia is, therefore, shaped by several dynamics. *First*, the experience of, for example, a diagnosis with dementia which society assumes to be 'catastrophic' is experienced as threatening to an individual's biography. However, through processes such as 'searching for meaning' there is the opportunity for the impact of the disruption to the person's life story to be minimised. These concepts of biography and life story narrative thread into the *second* issue in which risk has a dual positive and negative nature (as enhancing quality of life and as threatening safety). However, the dual nature of risk is in itself an inadequate understanding of an individual's experiences when living with the disabling effect of societies, which can restrict choice and decision making. As a result, the *third* issue concerns the contradictory way in which risk is used to promote both safety and autonomy. This tension in the deployment of 'risk' fuels, and is reflexively fuelled by a *fourth* issue: the contested and ever-changing location of responsibility and risk expertise. The dynamics of theory, policy and practice have a profound influence on the experience of people with dementia and their families, and need further analysis if we are to better enable people to live positively with dementia.

As seen, there are many different ways of understanding the concept of risk, but at its heart are issues of uncertainty of future outcomes from actions. It very often suggests negative outcomes yet positive risk taking is often admired and is recognised as being essential to a rewarding engagement with life. Risk is culturally embedded, meaning different things to different people and in different societies and contexts. For example, in dementia care, as with other areas of enduring health and social care, there are marked differences between the dominant knowledge of professional and lay people resulting in competing and different priorities in managing care. However, 'risk' in a formalised sense is primarily a preoccupation of countries which have highly regulated health and social care systems. It may be, therefore, less culturally embedded in developing countries. Indeed, in everyday life we are always negotiating risk in a less formalised way.

Douglas (1990) provides a very useful definition of risk: 'the probability of an event occurring combined with the magnitude of losses or gains that would be entailed' (p.2). This provides a balanced definition of risk which helps us to see the attractions of taking risks (such as personal fulfilment, challenge, excitement) as well as the common understanding of risk as something that suggests danger, harm and threat. There are a wide variety of ways in which individuals and groups make sense of risk. *Positive risk taking* or *risk-benefit assessment* are terms that have been promoted to ensure that the wellbeing and autonomy of the person with dementia is taken into account explicitly as well as focusing on any need for protection from physical harm (Nuffield Council on Bioethics 2009).

The importance of exploring these issues in relation to dementia has never been more pressing. In the UK the Alzheimer's Society (2007) has suggested that the numbers of people with dementia will rise from 700,000 in 2007 to 940,110 by 2021, an increase of 38 per cent over the next 15 years. This mirrors a world-wide increase in the prevalence of people experincing dementia. Such a rise will undoubtedly place additional demands on health and social care agencies, a demand that will only increase as the policy imperative of earlier detection and diagnosis of dementia comes to fruition (Department of Health 2009).

OUR BACKGROUND

We have worked together over several years with a shared interest in developing services and practices for people living with dementia through research and practice development. One focus of our work has been on how the concept of risk shapes people's lives and the way that practitioners relate to people living with dementia. In particular, we have been part of an international research network on risk in ageing populations (Clarke *et al.* 2006). This network has allowed us to explore these ideas with a wide range of colleagues.

We each bring different experiences to this book: Charlotte Clarke as a general nurse who worked with older people and people with dementia, and now professor of nursing practice development research; Heather Wilkinson as a social scientist with a particular interest in people with dementia and a learning disability, and now director of research; John Keady as a community psychiatric nurse who worked with people with dementia and their families, and now professor of older people's mental health nursing, a position he holds jointly with an NHS Mental Health Foundation Trust; Catherine Gibb as a speech and language therapist and now senior lecturer.

The ideas that we express in this book are based on our experiences in clinical practice, educational activities and in particular on several research studies that we have carried out (details are in the Appendix). We have used these studies in a general way in this book to illustrate some of the issues around risk assessment and risk management. They include:

- a study into the experiences of carers of people with dementia based on interview data (the Carer Study)

- a study of risk construction and management in dementia care, based on an organisational survey, interviews with people with dementia and their carers and collaborative learning groups with practitioners (the Risk Study)

- an action research study into continence management in acute dementia care environments (the Continence Study)

- a study of risk construction by people with dementia living in disadvantaged communities in South Africa (the South African Study).

PRINCIPLES AND AIM

There are a few principles or key messages which we want to highlight and which we will return to throughout the book.

1. The 'problem' of dementia is not a problem which belongs to individuals, and it is important to refocus away from people with dementia to allow us to understand the interrelationship they have with the wider community and its impact on them.

2. As a practitioner, risk is something that is ever-present and which shapes your professional assessment and decision making. It is something that can make us apprehensive (we may feel we need to 'cover our backs') and uncertain about how we might support people to 'take risks'.

3. Risk does not in itself mean something that is negative or harmful, although we acknowledge that it is very often viewed in this way. Think of risk as a chance of something. This chance may have harmful consequences but it may alternatively have positive consequences which may enhance quality of life.

4. Removing risk totally from someone's life is not possible or desirable because it would compromise quality of life; but risk can be negotiated and managed to make sure that harmful consequences are minimised and positive consequences are maximised.

5. Very often different people will view something in different ways leading to multiple perspectives on risk. In such circumstances, it is essential that the person with dementia is supported to express their own perspective and their choices are enabled where possible. As such, risk management is a process of negotiation.

6. The ideas and values that we explore in this book are relevant in all settings, including residential care homes and community environments.

We have one primary aim for this book – to create the opportunity for you to think about your own position and practice in relation to risk and the position that others take. We have included 'Think about' sections in the book which invite you to pause and reflect on your own views and practice, either by yourself or through discussion with your colleagues.

Part II
Different Views on Risk

Chapter 2

Living with Dementia
Living with Risk

INTRODUCTION

This chapter explores one of the most challenging aspects of viewing risk, and one that has a major impact on our management of it – that different people have different views on what is important and what a risk is. In this chapter, we consider why there are different viewpoints and how they came about. In particular, we focus on the viewpoint of people with dementia to try to illustrate how they are continually engaged in a process of trying to make their priorities and risk management known in order to live well with dementia.

PERCEPTIONS AND DIFFERING VIEWS

The National Institute for Health and Clinical Excellence (NICE) and the Social Care Institute for Excellence (SCIE) guideline *Dementia: Supporting People with Dementia and their Carers in Health and Social Care* (NICE clinical practice guideline 42; NICE/SCIE 2007) promoted a biopsychosocial approach to understanding dementia and acting as a platform for intervention. The biopsychosocial approach has led to an emphasis on modifying the course of dementia through processes such as early/timely diagnosis, assessment and cognitive rehabilitation, with treatment including prescription of the anti-dementia drugs where they are indicated. The biopsychosocial approach also places significant emphasis on understanding the personal experience of living with the condition and how the person constructs, and re-constructs, the reality of their day-to-day life. Since the late 1980s, a major proponent of the psychosocial approach in dementia care was Tom Kitwood who defined the construct of personhood as a 'standing or status bestowed upon one human being, by others, in the context of a relationship and social being' (Kitwood 1997, p.8). An increasing body of research has explored the experiences of living with a dementia, whether with the diagnosis or as a carer, and studies have progressed from a focus in the 1980s and 1990s on the burdens of caring to research which focuses more on the interrelationship underpinning care giving and receiving (Gates 2000; Todres and Galvin 2006), and more recently by Nolan *et al.* (2008) where these interrelationships become the focal point for understanding the dynamics of living with dementia.

The knowledge base that is used in dementia care is largely drawn from experience acquired in practice working with people with dementia and their families, and through education and learning about the models and research evidence which underpins practices. Increasingly, it is research, or evidence-based practice, which professionals are encouraged to base practice on. However, this can be hard to fit in to our experiences and is certainly not necessarily the way in which people with dementia and carers view their needs. In relation to experiences of risk, Douglas (1994) emphasises how evidence-based practice ignores the complex cultural and political aspects of risk. In the following section we draw on research in which carers of people with dementia were interviewed about this topic (the Carer Study; Clarke 1997).

While practitioners draw on research evidence and generalised beliefs acquired during their training, socialisation and clinical experience, family carers have a detailed experience of the person with dementia as an individual, and of their particular circumstances (as of course do people with dementia themselves). In this sense, people with dementia and families are more concerned with the social meaning of the condition than they are in its cause and prognosis. As a result, people with dementia and carers have to negotiate the involvement of practitioners so that it fits into their own concerns and lives.

Let us take the example of Dorothy who cares for her husband with dementia. In the following quote she describes how, despite the challenges of the changing nature of their relationship, the provision of respite care, she feels, does not necessarily meet her needs:

> I don't feel like that I want him to go on holiday (respite care). I feel like I want him to be in the house, 'cause sometimes he's good company you know, he makes you laugh. One time he made me cry a lot but now, I'm getting used to him altogether now.

The reciprocity within a care relationship means that both the carer and the person with dementia are working towards keeping some stability, continuity and sense of the normal in their lives. Health and social care interventions, or others outside that caring relationship, rarely provide validation of the relationship as at all 'normal', and so while interventions may support the continuance of the relationship (through supporting someone to live at home as long as possible for example) they also throw a spotlight on the abnormal by focusing on the illness more than on getting on with life. Accordingly, this can have a negative impact on those trying to see their lives as having some normality.

These tensions relate to time, person and problem. Practitioners are largely orientated to future events, emphasising the problematic prognosis of people with dementia. Family carers know of the past person, who now happens to have dementia, and interpret their future in relation to that knowledge, seeking to value the individual and minimise the intrusiveness of the dementia. Practitioners do not usually have any knowledge and experience of the person with dementia before they were diagnosed and so they have been denied access to this very individual and 'person knowledge' that the family carer and the individual themselves base their day-to-day life on. For practitioners, their experiences with the individual commence in the present and are not building on a past relationship. Their knowledge lies in an awareness of others who have had dementia, others who have progressed through the course of the illness. They are therefore denied the opportunity to relate to the person with dementia as they once were, but may instead relate to the person with dementia as someone facing continual decline and cognitive disability. These issues of different time frames, knowledge of the person and understanding of the problem can lead directly to different perceptions of risk between people with dementia, carers and practitioners. For example, Sarah allowed her father, who had dementia, to leave their home on his own regularly even though he often got lost because she felt that he needed that sense of freedom and self-determination. Indeed, in similar situations, practitioners may see this as a risk behaviour in need of limiting and modifying.

Table 2.1 A comparison of risk knowledges

Person with dementia perspective	Family carer perspective	Professional carer perspective
Intimate knowledge of personal history and aspirations	Specific knowledge of person	General knowledge of dementia
Knowledge of individual need	Knowledge of individual need	Knowledge of the needs of people with dementia
Seek to normalise and assimilate situation	Seek to normalise situation	Seek to pathologise situation
Seek to disconfirm expected trajectory of decline	Seek to disconfirm expected trajectory of decline	Seek to confirm expected trajectory of decline
Personal knowledge claims	Personal/political knowledge claims	Evidence-based knowledge claims
Values/meaning discourse	Values/meaning discourse	Facts discourse

Source: Adapted from Clarke and Heyman 1998

There are, then, three knowledge bases in action – the family carer's knowledge of the person, the practitioner's knowledge of the disease that is dementia, and critically the knowledge held by the person with dementia (see Table 2.1). These knowledge bases are not held exclusively and, to some extent, attempts are made to learn of each other's knowledge, such as through life histories. Although at times these knowledges may be in conflict, they each guide the practices of the carer, be they a family carer or practitioner.

Think about – Use Table 2.1 to think about a carer of someone with dementia who you know. Where are there some gaps between the carer's and the professional's expectations and goals? Why is this? What can you do to overcome these gaps?

Even when the person with dementia requires care beyond the knowledge and ability of the family carer, a 'normal' life is not relinquished. Their life together is redefined into another normality which embraces the difficulties concerning living with dementia. Bury (1991) refers to this process of redefinition as biographical disruption and accommodation – an untoward event becomes assimilated into a redefined future and in itself shapes people's perceptions of their present and past. For example, Ian sees no reason why his mother's confusion and continence difficulties should preclude her from involvement in their financial affairs, or deny her the opportunity to go out on day trips. This may contrast with the perspective of practitioners whose purpose it is to assess and in so doing, seek out 'the abnormal', or the failings, in the person. Thus, the lives of the person with dementia and their family carer become relatively problem-orientated, dominated by what is wrong in their lives rather than what is ordinary and normal.

Any relationship exists as an interactive process and is never a static state. In professional care, services need to fully recognise and acknowledge this shifting dynamic of a relationship since it has a profound effect on those being supported and indeed on their relationship with us. For example, family carers may be reluctant to let others know of the individual's failing cognitive ability, protecting them from the social reaction of stigma, but in so doing also denying themselves and the (undiagnosed) person with dementia access to health and social interventions and help. In the Carer Study, Christine, for example, described the pre-diagnostic phase as 'a traumatic experience' because she was torn between accessing help and being loyal to her husband with dementia who 'didn't want people to think he was an idiot'. The wishes of the person with dementia may be a key determinant in the acceptance or refusal of service intervention by the family carer.

The dominant professional approach to dementia care, emphasising the abnormal, the pathological and the prognosis of deterioration, undermines the relationship-orientated approach to caregiving. It does, however, offer structure and some meaning to events and allows planning to be made for future problems, although arguably thereby contributing to their creation (Clarke and Keady 1996). The approach governed by normalisation, however, is grounded in the relationship of the person with dementia and the family carer, and is woven into the fabric of their lives. It operates in relation to the past, the person and the problem-free. These differences are highlighted too by Mitchell and Glendinning (2007) who explore the relationship between risk and a 'normal' life, and highlight the differing assumptions of family carers and practitioners which inform care.

Family carers and people with dementia want, and work towards, maintaining a relationship with someone who is important to their lives, and in which disease and problems can be kept minimally intrusive. For many this is achieved with little or no professional intervention. However, when interventions are necessary, it will best support the aspirations of the individual and carer if it acknowledges their knowledge base as at least equal, but different, to a professional knowledge base. An effective care intervention will make careful use of both these knowledge bases, with the aim of allowing someone to live well with dementia and fulfilling the needs of the relationship between the family and then person with dementia. Practitioners should be encouraged to look to the person with dementia's past and cultural context instead of holding a perception of the person's future, and to see freedom from problems instead of 'the problematic'. Galvin, Todres and Richardson (2005) describe a single case study in a paper co-written with a spouse carer of someone with dementia, which identifies the 'intimate' carer as a mediator between the private experiences of someone with dementia and the public nature of health and social care systems.

We also need to think about what the implications of having a diagnosis of dementia itself means for the individual and how society's beliefs about the diagnosis can in themselves be a threat to people who have dementia. The effects of labelling people were discussed by Illiffe and Manthorpe (2004) – they identify that early diagnosis and labelling someone as a person with dementia can impact on their self-esteem and identity. Early diagnosis risks devaluing the mental capacity of the individual and introduces inappropriate assumptions about reduced competence. Furthermore, the individual may themselves come to question their own mental capacity, further compromising their self-esteem.

It is essential that we take diversity and equality into account in risk assessment and management. There is little written about cultural diversity in dementia care, yet in other areas we know that culture can have a risk-magnifying effect (for example, people who are black being stopped by police to a greater extent than white people). Daker-White *et al.* (2002), in their study of carers of people with dementia who are Asian or African Caribbean, did not find any real difference in how risk was viewed compared to white carers but they do highlight the problems of communication and language and the importance of culturally sensitive services.

DEMENTIA CARE AND RISK IN DEVELOPING COUNTRIES

Within health and social care, risk is predominantly a concern of the more developed world, where health and social care systems are more sophisticated and regulated. We have already seen that even for the Western world, the notion of risk assessment and management within dementia care is not well defined and still being negotiated.

This means that for developing countries where dementia care is still in its infancy, the notion of risk itself has barely received an acknowledgement. However, it is crucial that we give some attention to risk in relation to other countries and other cultures. Risks faced by people with dementia and their families are most often defined by services and a focus on safety and security, which may result in service provision that is not fully negotiated with the person with dementia and possibly inclined to be unduly protective and neglectful of cultural influences.

There are four major global shifts which influence the experiences of all people with dementia and which enhance or compromise someone's quality of life (Clarke *et al.* 2006):

- an increasingly ageing population (rising to 1000 million older people by 2020) and with it an associated rise in age-related long-term conditions

- the double burden of communicable disease and long-term conditions in developing countries, and the growing proportion of people living with a long-term condition in more developed countries (18 million in the UK alone)

- the growth of culturally sensitive ethical regard which heralds a challenge to the ideologically loaded concept of quality of care

- expanding social and cultural notions of risk will challenge the location and nature of risk expertise, creating space for self-management.

The increasing ageing of the population leads to an increased incidence of dementia, especially in the least developed and developing regions of the world (Kalaria *et al.* 2008). Although an estimated 66 per cent of people with dementia in the world live in developing countries, far less research is conducted and fewer resources are allocated to the disease and its management in developing countries, compared with the developed world (Prince *et al.* 2004). Current epidemiology figures are not accurate due to lack of awareness of dementia and inadequate diagnostic assessment in these regions. In developing countries there is little or no long-term care for people with dementia, therefore they are much more reliant on families to provide for their needs. Current research indicates that, particularly in parts of Latin America, and in India, a disturbingly high proportion of people with dementia lack the basic necessities for life, such as food (Kalaria *et al.* 2008). In such circumstances risk assessment and management in dementia would look very different to that of the Western world.

A study of dementia care in South Africa

To illustrate some of these international and cultural issues, we will draw on a small study that was done in South Africa (the South African Study) and which aimed to understand some of the cross-cultural issues relating to risk and dementia (more information on this research is given in the Appendix, p.115). The stark contrast between the situations of people with dementia living in the first world compared with the third world is highlighted where different cultures live side by side, such as South Africa. Despite living under the same government, the social circumstances of a black person with dementia living in an informal settlement are very different to those of a wealthy white person living in the suburbs. Within the multi-lingual, multi-ethnic South African context such issues are exacerbated by historical apartheid divisions.

In 2002, South Africans aged 60 years and over constituted 6 per cent of the population, projected to increase to 14 per cent by 2050 (UN 2007). An epidemiology of dementia is not yet available in South Africa for many reasons, among which are:

- a low priority given to the mental health care of older persons in the public health sector

- a lack of culturally appropriate cognitive function screening instruments for older black South Africans

- the relatively low proportion of cognitively impaired older black people who seek support from the health care system (Ferreira and Makoni 1999).

The research was undertaken in the Cape Town metropole in South Africa, and involved the following three non-governmental organisations, based in three areas of Cape Town. Interviews were conducted with people living with dementia, and a focus group was also conducted in each of the organisations to explore each community's understanding of dementia, and the meaning of risk in the context of dementia.

1. *Grandmothers Against Poverty and AIDS*, Khayelitsha. This organisation is run by and works with older women from the local township, which comprises predominantly black South Africans. Khayelitsha is a low socio-economic area approximately 20 kilometres outside Cape Town. It is home to approximately 850,000 people. Homes in Khayelitsha are either brick structures or shacks or a combination of both.

2. *Rehoboth Age Exchange* – part of *City Mission, South Africa*. Day care and service programmes serve the most vulnerable physically and mentally frail older persons with a special focus on stroke, Alzheimer's disease and other dementias. At the time of the research (2005–2006) this was the only dedicated day care service for persons with Alzheimer's disease and other dementias in a poor community in South Africa. It is based in Hanover Park, where the majority of the community are mixed race ('coloured') South Africans.

3. The Rondebosch support group of *Dementia South Africa*. This group serves a majority white South African population, from a wide area of south-east Cape Town, and mainly supports family members caring for a relative with dementia.

For all the people with dementia who were interviewed, their family carers and professionals, the high level of crime prevalent in South Africa was perceived as a great risk. This leads to a high level of fear, especially where people with dementia are on their own at home during the day:

> the crime is increased, so I think if they wandered or anything they would not be safe…in these areas it's a

big risk, so you can't you feel safe about them wandering or even leaving them alone at home if they are even mild dementia. (carer)

Abuse and neglect were also recognised as a big problem for people with dementia, especially those living in townships. This was often linked with financial abuse, exacerbated by high levels of unemployment and related poverty. Often the pension of the person with dementia was the only income into the household (the equivalent of about £80 a month), leading to frequent financial exploitation by family members: 'a daughter put her mother out of her own house... She's got dementia...they put her out, got her house up for sale... Someone was drawing her pension...' (carer).

Levels of awareness of dementia were generally low, especially in black and coloured communities: 'People aren't identifying and aren't taking them to the doctor because they think they're just going mad' (carer). In Khayelitsha, participants explained how there is still much superstition around the symptoms of dementia, often leading to a person being labelled as a 'witch' with consequent implications for inclusion (and often exclusion) from the community. A related issue is the denial of rights of the people with dementia: 'You still get people not recognising that this is a human being, this person is to be respected and this person has got as much right as you have...' (professional).

For people with dementia and their families in South Africa there is a lack of provision of the support that is taken for granted in the UK – day care, financial support, medical care, social care. Even for families with private medical insurance, there are few support options for the people with dementia themselves and the family. Dementia has only recently been recognised politically, but it is hoped that the 2006 Older Persons Act (Republic of South Africa (RSA) 2006) has begun to address this situation.

Think about – What are the cultural aspects of being older for people you work with? How does this influence their understanding of risk?

THE VIEWS OF PEOPLE WITH DEMENTIA AND CARERS

Let us now focus on the perspective of people with dementia and their carers and how they accept and work with risk as part of everyday life. In this section, we are going to follow the stories and experiences of four people with dementia in the UK to see how risk impacted on their lives and why the ways in which the risk was managed could make a difference to their everyday lives. This work draws on our research into risk construction and management in dementia care (the Risk Study, see Appendix, p.114).

We have taken this case study or story approach so that the experiences of the different people – the person with dementia, professional, family carer – can be included. We see into a little of the lives of Margaret, Mary, Jack and Martin to illustrate process and change. The processes and changes experienced by people allow us to see how an understanding of the issues and possibilities of risk assessment and management shift over time and can inform a more balanced decision-making process. Margaret, Mary, Jack and Martin were four people who were involved with us in a research study into risk management (along with 51 others). We interviewed each of them up to three times, and invited them to nominate a family carer and one of their practitioners for us to approach to interview too.

- *Margaret* lives on her own in sheltered accommodation. She is in her early sixties and has two children. Margaret knows she has had dementia for about three years and has other mental and physical health care difficulties. Margaret nominated her daughter Sarah and her occupational therapist to participate in the study.

- *Martin* lives with his wife Jane in a very remote rural area. Martin is in his early eighties and otherwise well, although Jane has some physical health difficulties. Martin nominated Jane and his community practitioner to participate in the study.

- *Jack* lives with his wife Kath in their own home and has day care each week. Jack is in his late seventies and also has other mental and physical health care difficulties. Jack nominated Kath and his community psychiatric nurse to participate in the study.

- *Mary* lives with her partner Peter in their own home and attended a hospital-based day centre. Mary nominated Peter and one of the day centre staff to participate in the study.

We use these real life examples to explore five key areas that were 'contested territories' for people when living with dementia (Clarke *et al.* 2010). These five contested territories of everyday life are: friendships, smoking, going out, domestic arrangements and occupation and activity. By exploring these contested territories we are not proposing that risk be completely removed. Acknowledging issues such as 'whose risk?' and how decisions are negotiated and thought through, we can gain a better understanding of the process of risk assessment and management. This helps us have a realistic idea of situations faced by people with dementia.

It is also important to acknowledge the impact of personal histories and biographical aspects of people's lives so that we can see individuals' purpose and make sense of the contested territories. Through this, we can better support the maintenance of the person with dementia's sense of self, support decision making, and create purpose in people's lives.

Assessing and managing risk in a way that takes into account how these contested territories are formed and worked out will support care that is person-centred, and moreover respectful of the relationships that contribute to maintaining the individual's sense of self and purpose.

The contested territory of friendships

Mary used the friendships in her life to achieve two things. First, to relate to people with similar experiences as a way of making sense of her position (as also illustrated in relation to smoking below): 'We can all have a laugh together about the things that we've all done, you know, and it seems to lift the load' (Mary). This was recognised too by her practitioner and by her partner Peter: 'So they are all in the same boat and she realises she is not alone anymore.'

Second, friendship enables Mary to maintain a sense of self and identity: 'I still see my friends and I enjoy going out with them. I feel human after that, when I have actually been out with friends.' In particular, Mary draws a contrast between being 'out with the girls' and being out with Peter when 'It is always "Now don't do this" or "Don't do that…" or "No…you'll not like that"'. None-the-less, Mary recognises her dependence on her friends when they are out and its impact on their time together:

> I am not allowed to go out now unless I have one of my family with me. Whereas before I could go and ring up one of my friends. And I can understand that they'll say 'Oh, I've got something planned'. It's because, although we have been very good friends for a long time, is that they don't want to have to take the risk of taking me out on their own. And I agree with them. Because if anything were to happen to me they would feel it was their fault. Well it isn't, it's me! (Mary)

Mary illustrates the role that others play in another of the key contested territories, that of 'getting out'. Getting out is important to her, but is something she states she is 'not allowed' to do alone, and that is problematic for her friends. Martin recognised too that, as his dementia progressed, when he went fishing his friend was 'always on the lookout for me'.

Martin often felt tongue-tied in conversations, which frustrated him in his friendships:

> I think most people I know understand, and will wait for it to come out or I say 'Oh forget it!' [laughs]. Jane's [his wife] got to help me with a lot of words of course, but I think that's the worst, because it upsets you, you're not one of the boys again, at all you see. Whereas you should be talking to people about the old days and telling them all about it, I can't do it. (Martin)

However, Jane is starting to feel that their friends are less inclined to meet up, as in the quote below, and is protective of Martin being exposed as unable to manage larger public events with friends:

> I'm beginning to feel, we have quite a lot of lovely friends and relatives, and there's the odd one or two that…an

excuse not to stop long because he takes so long to tell people his stories and he gets all confused that I think some people get a little bit bored or intolerant of it. (Jane)

One of the other people with dementia, Margaret, identifies the need for a balance in being with friends and relatives: 'A friend comes over once a week, we go out for a meal, that's enough. I don't want to be with people all the time, I like to be on my own.' Margaret has experienced a contraction of her friendships as a result of her own withdrawal from activities (including voluntary work and as a counsellor) and as friends have died, resulting in an impoverished experience for herself:

> I miss sort of stimulating conversation...and I miss meeting interesting people and all, I miss that I must say, I don't very often meet interesting people now... When I was in [voluntary work]...there was quite a lot of interesting women, and when I used to go to counselling I had a few interesting friends and they've all gone. ...I've had a few friends died as well, close friends have died. ...I talk to people on the net, which has been a life saver really. (Margaret)

Margaret's friends were seen by her daughter Sarah, the main carer, as an important support network which together with service involvement 'makes it easier for both of us and then our relationship is less fraught' (Sarah). Both Sarah and Margaret's nominated practitioner wish she had more confidence to be involved with her friends and join in social activities.

Think about – What is the importance of knowing who is part of important and supportive relationships? How can these be maintained? Where is the risk in not maintaining these? How can these friendships be sustained if someone moves into a care home?

The contested territory of smoking

For Mary, smoking was an important part of her daily life. It provided simultaneously an explanation for her stroke-related dementia and was, paradoxically, also a source of comfort:

> I feel that man upstairs [God] has played a rotten joke on me by giving me this disease I've got and I can't get rid of. Other people would say 'Well you shouldn't smoke', but that's the only pleasure I've got, it calms me down. (Mary)

Smoking was also a key feature of Mary's social network activities and through these she made sense of her current situation:

> [Smoking is] one of the reasons why I come to places like this [day centre]. It gives me other female company and we can have a laugh, we can discuss things. Sometimes I make them laugh. I come out with some daft things. …yes, we do talk you know about, there's no restriction. There's about four of us like to go outside for a cigarette but there's a special place now where we can sit indoors. I can have a cigarette and discuss things. When you hear some of the tales other people tell you, you think to yourself straightaway 'Oh, well there's not just me'. (Mary)

Moreover, smoking was a territory of her life that was highly contested by her partner Peter, something that Mary was well aware of and she had adapted her behaviour to avoid his censure:

> He gets on at me, so I normally do it [smoking] when he goes shopping or I might at night when he might have gone out. (Mary)

Peter was anxious to explain that he not only regarded smoking as one of the causes of her stroke but that he had reason to be concerned for her welfare from continuing to smoke:

> She's burning her jumpers, because she has jumpers with holes in you know. Dressing gown, full of holes here. I

says 'What happened?' Shall I get it? [Peter leaves the room to get Mary's dressing gown.] You see the way she has left these burns in it?

[Interviewer – 'Oh dear, yeah. All around the back as well.']

That's what I worry about. And that's the risk that when I go out that she sets fire to this place. (Peter)

In seeking to manage this contested area of Mary's life, Peter was becoming increasingly vigilant and reluctant to leave her alone for more than half an hour. It is interesting that, when this was discussed with the practitioner, smoking did not appear in the analysis of perceived and assessed risk factors.

Think about – What are the pros and cons of Mary smoking? Are there strategies that can minimise risk?

The contested territory of going out

Going out, whether on foot or by car, was invariably a territory that was contested and which raised many challenges for people with dementia and those who cared for them. For example, as well as smoking (described above), going out was another activity disputed between Mary and Peter and which she perceived as necessary to retaining her identity:

I miss doing things most women do, go shopping. ... now and again I sneak out... I don't tell Peter because he'll go off it. He doesn't like me going out unless there was someone with me. I mean everybody in the street knows me, even in the shop, but 'If you want something you tell me and I'll bring it up' and I think 'Well, I'm sitting here doing nothing, I could be around and back'

> but he'll not have it. …I think he's frightened in case I
> take a wrong turning and I don't know where I am. But
> I cannot possibly take a wrong turning where we live.
> 'What do you want to go in there? You should have told
> me I would have brought it in' and I think 'Oh man, give
> it a rest'. (Mary)

This contested activity of going out was recognised by Mary's practitioner:

> Going out with her partner was difficult because she can't
> walk very far…she hasn't got the muscle strength. So I
> felt that her choices were limited and most of the choices
> in what she wanted were being made by Peter, her partner.
> …so we talked about how having a wheelchair would
> enable her to maintain her ability. (Mary's practitioner)

Margaret, like Mary, has mobility difficulties that are not related to dementia. Margaret, however, is reluctant to go outside her home:

> I don't go out very much, I don't go out at all on my
> own… I went down to the dentist yesterday, but I got a
> taxi there and back and I don't like it, I hate it, I feel a bit
> vulnerable, but my sister takes us and my daughter takes
> us… (Margaret)

One of the reasons that Margaret dislikes going out is that she hates relying on other people: 'I hate depending on other people, and you're asking people to do things for you.'

Having experienced her own mother with dementia 'wandering', Margaret joked: 'at least I cannot wander very far because I've not got the mobility [laughs]'. Margaret's practitioner feels that she is 'more cautious than I'd like her to be. …go out a little bit more. She's very fearful about going out by herself now'. Margaret's daughter, Sarah, however, recognises her mother's reluctance to go out as a concern which she links to the contested territory of friendship: 'She just refuses to go anywhere without anybody so she's very isolated.'

The part that going out plays in maintaining friendships was also experienced by Jack who enjoyed amateur dramatics and had hoped to transport his fellow actors:

> As far as the driving was concerned, I lost my orientation. I kept getting lost in other words. So I decided and I was advised, by that time, my medical condition was more obvious or evident, so I was told I shouldn't drive. …I was on the point of getting a minibus to take people… but I just had to give that up and a lot of my colleagues, if you could call them that, were disappointed that I had to give all this up. (Jack)

Jack also experienced some attention by staff in the day centre regarding his mobility and movements, which he resented a little:

> They're inclined to be a little bit fussy in the centre that I go to. If somebody doesn't stick to the path sort of thing. I mean with the best of intentions, they are anxious that you don't do anything by which you'll injure yourself. When I first went there I was a bit piqued because I didn't think I was that bad…
>
> [Interviewer – 'So what kind of things do they discourage you from doing there?']
>
> Well stepping out of the building. I wanted to get some fresh air. Anyway, they found somewhere I could sit, which solved that problem. …oh they're very exact about the way I walk, the way I use my walker because I'm inclined to cross my hands or something silly like that or just put it one-handed and they stop me doing that but they do it in the best, in a good humoured way. (Jack)

For Martin, driving remained an important part of his life since he and his wife lived in a very remote area without access to shops or other facilities without driving. Although his wife Jane drives, she felt that to stop driving would be very hard for him: 'Oh I think it would kill him if they [took away] the driving! Not kill him but I think that would be terrible! I think he'd deteriorate if he couldn't drive' (Jane). The difficulties of this were recognised by Martin's practitioner:

> I think she's quite anxious about what happens if he stops driving as well, because they live in an isolated place... He goes up the [motorway] doesn't he? [laughter]...must be horrific if you've got even a slight memory problem, it's bad enough when you haven't...they've always done it. (Martin's practitioner)

Think about – What are the different risks for each individual? How can these be negotiated?

The contested territory of domestic arrangements

It was over domestic arrangements as a contested territory that there appeared to be most disputes over relinquishing (former) responsibilities. These disputes demonstrated ways in which people with dementia sought to retain their independence and sense of themselves. Mary illustrates this in the following descriptions of how she and Peter have renegotiated their roles in the home, and the impact of this on her sense of autonomy. She describes Peter as having to 'put the "no go" face on' when he steps in to stop her doing something. As Mary went on to explain:

> I'm not allowed to do anything in the house. I've always had someone who comes to do my housework. It's not because I'm lazy, it's because I haven't got the power to do it. If I did try to do it by myself well I'd make a, excuse the language, a hell of a mess. ...sometimes, the odd times when I've washed up, because Peter does that, I've managed the washing, and dried them, but I put them back all in the wrong places. So he's had to sort

that out. 'Will you please leave that alone?', and I feel as though I'm not wanted. (Mary)

[Interviewer – Before you were ill were you the one who made the decisions…is that a big change?]

Yeah. I decided when we went food shopping and what we would have for a meal, we could eat out or we could come home, anything like that, or if there was anyone in the family that wasn't very well it was me who said 'You'll have to get some flowers and go and visit them. We will have to'. But now he does all of the things like that. (Mary)

Peter concurs with these changes in their domestic roles: 'I took Mary over and I'm doing all her thinking now' (Peter). Although doing the majority of the domestic activities now, Peter describes how 'the problem now is watching, wondering what she's doing now you know, mislaying things' (Peter). Mary's practitioner described how, through attendance at the day centre, Mary now had a renewed interest in her home, was choosing how to redecorate it, and had a wider range of things to converse with Peter about:

So she is decision making. That was our greatest fear when she came here was that Peter was taking over her decision making. And that's the last straw if she is someone with a strong personality where someone is not allowing me to make my decisions, it makes you feel childish. (verbatim, Mary's practitioner)

Margaret's daughter Sarah was also faced with making decisions about when to step in to help her mother: 'I worry when she cleans the fish tank out because it's great big buckets of water…but at the same time, they're part of normal things to do, so you don't want to say "Oh no".' Similarly, when Margaret's practitioner was asked what was seen to be the most important things for Margaret, she replied: 'Being able to do her own thing, when she wants, how she wants, not somebody coming in and managing her, her life.'

Margaret has also relinquished domestic activities which she had previously found satisfying and fulfilling:

> I've stopped cooking, I used to cook for the family and I can't do that anymore because I've scalded myself so many times… I forget to put the gas off, I turn the wrong lever and I've set light to a couple of tea towels… I used to love cooking, I really did. I enjoyed it, baking and making meals and things like that, I was sort of known for all my cooking. Now I can't, I live out of packets. I'm slowly getting rid of things out of the cupboard… it's hard to give the things up, the cupboard's still full of cooking things. (Margaret)

Jack had also relinquished cooking activities: 'He doesn't do any of that now… I think it was just something that happened. He just wasn't able to do it so it just wasn't done anymore' (Jack's wife Kath). As a result Jack's practitioner recognised that he was vulnerable to his wife's poor health and possible inability to look after Jack.

Margaret also highlighted her diminishing financial control ('I forget to pay') but her reluctance to stop having access to credit: 'I don't feel I'm ready to give [credit card] up yet.' Unlike Margaret, Jack's diminishing financial control had resulted in debt and he no longer managed the domestic finances: 'I mean when they discovered (the debt) it was quite a shock to the system' (Kath).

One aspect of domestic arrangements is dealing with medical appointments, and at times relatives described needing to advocate for the person with dementia and to accompany them on medical appointments. Margaret's daughter Sarah described how her mother 'likes someone to fight her corner sometimes, and then it irritates her that people have to fight her corner'.

In Martin's life, he had relinquished different aspects, including the role he had assumed previously of organising holidays for a group of friends, and day-to-day communication and finances:

> I used to do all the work…but it's all, had to turn it over to her [Jane, his wife] you see – who's really good, I think she's far better than me actually I ever was… I used

> to take [relatives and friends on holiday] and I used to
> hold everything, the kitty and everything and get them
> on the bus or whatever it was, 'Come on, this is it' and
> that type of thing and everything like that, well that's
> gone now. (Martin)

The care that the person with dementia showed for their relative remained strong, and was a particular concern for Martin: 'I'm worried about her [his wife Jane] more than anything, that she's been very poorly, because this is the second time round you know, and I don't want her to do things, I'd rather let the bloody house fall to pieces...' Martin's practitioner described how Jane keeps him involved and active in household matters: 'I think he does a lot for her, and I think she does bully him into doing it as well. She doesn't let him sit there and she doesn't wait on him hand and foot so he is part of the household as well.'

Think about – What are the risks relating to domestic arrangements – are they actual or perceived risks? What strategies can be used to help this situation?

The contested territory of occupation and activity

Margaret is a former nurse, and now at 60 years old, had spent time in several roles since leaving nursing, each of which she has had to leave as her health has deteriorated. As a result she has had to adapt to frequent changes of activity, and with each change has had to address feeling unable to continue. At present, Margaret is enjoying making cards which are sold at craft fairs. Each of these changes addresses the need for Margaret to have a sense of purpose in her life. She describes how she has 'just sort of substituted things':

> [when I left nursing] It was horrible for a little while and
> I felt useless...started to do voluntary work...and then
> did a counselling diploma and did voluntary counselling

for up to about three years...so I was quite busy...when I had to stop I felt useless.

[Interviewer – 'What led to you stopping the counselling?']

Well, because I couldn't remember people's stories you know, I got mixed up with them and I mean it's quite stressful counselling... Then I set up a library (for a woman's health group), do the books and things, but then that even got, because I got mixed up I didn't know where things were, I didn't know which books I'd done and which I hadn't and I got my system mixed up so I gave that up... I felt a bit down again, useless... (Margaret)

Her daughter Sarah associates these occupation changes with constant changes in her mother's social networks and friendships too. Although not mentioned by Margaret herself, Sarah does leave her children with Margaret regularly: 'I leave her grandchildren with her because one, it alleviates the fact that she feels useless. You know, she's now, she's great with the kids. Except [one of her children aged 8 years] who is going through that yak yak yak age and it does her head in...' (Sarah).

Think about – What are the different views of risk? What suggestions could you make to the people involved to help them understand each other's views?

EVERYDAY LIFE

The move to focus on ways in which people themselves live with dementia has brought an interest in day-to-day experiences. A diagnosis of dementia introduces an unfamiliar element into a familiar home, which is otherwise associated with notions of being a non-threatening environment, habitual routines and a place to be free from surveillance. Askham *et al.* (2007) describe how life for a person with dementia living at home is 'in constant danger of slipping towards the practices and life of a total institution' (p.21), which implies routinisation of activity, a level of surveillance of an individual's activities and behaviours and 'mortification of the self' (p.21), in which the dignity of the person is compromised.

In the Risk Study (see Appendix, 'Risk Construction and Management in Dementia Care' on p.114) of risk perception by people with dementia and carers, the everyday life of people with dementia was explored. We found that there were several areas of their lives which became places in which these different perceptions of risk were played out and which affected the way in which they were able to lead their lives (Clarke *et al.* 2010).

For people living with dementia, the implications are two-fold:

1. The everyday life of someone with dementia becomes an unstable structure with tension because the expectations of adult independence and established family life are confronted with the expectations of dementia as a disease and psychosocial entity. For example, Margaret describes how she has stopped cooking because of her forgetfulness yet it is an activity she enjoys and she is reluctant to discard the now unused food and cooking equipment.

2. Each member of the triad of person with dementia, family carer and practitioner seeks to form a bridge into each others' practice, recognising their need for each other but also their differences. For example, Mary, her partner Peter and her nominated practitioner all raised concern about how extensive Mary's own decision making should be.

The practices of 'everyday life' are a means of conceptualising the fluid way in which people live with a dementia. There are four core dimensions which arise from the contested territories of everyday life identified in the Risk Study by Clarke *et al.* (2010), and which render the territory as a place of purpose in the fluidity of lives which are being constantly redefined by the introduction of dementia into peoples' lives.

1. *Sense making.* One purpose of a contested territory is to provide an explanation for events, such as Mary's reference to smoking as both the cause of her stroke and her comfort in managing its consequences. In this way, Mary rationalises that to maintain her quality of life, smoking and going to the shops alone are actions which make sense. Margaret, however, made sense of having stopped cooking as she felt unsafe doing so, despite encouragement from others to maintain this interest.

2. *Maintaining self.* A second purpose of a contested territory is to maintain a sense of self. As dementia (or at least its social consequences) threatens an individual's awareness of themselves and their ability to express themselves, so the person with dementia retaliates by accessing activities which reinforce their identity. For example, Mary likes to maintain 'doing things most women do', and Martin regretted being unable to continue to organise holidays with his friends. This process may or may not be supported by a family carer or a practitioner: Jane, for example, was described as working to ensure that her husband Martin stayed involved in household activities. Both Jack and Martin were faced with contemplating stopping driving – but while Jack had stopped, Martin continued to drive and was supported to do so by his wife and practitioners. Crisp (1999) describes people with dementia as engaged in the process of 'defending, negotiating and reconstructing an identity for themselves' as they make sense of their diagnosis and their changing relationships with the people around them.

3. *Claiming and relinquishing decision making.* This third purpose of a contested territory is arguably the area of most conflict. It reflects the changing social and family positioning of the person with dementia in which their decision-making role is gradually adjusted. At times, decision making was relinquished voluntarily by the person with dementia. At other times, the family carer or indeed the practitioner assumed, or claimed, authority over decision-making processes, or sought to influence another's authority. For example, Mary's practitioner was concerned about the level of decision making claimed

by her partner Peter. Indeed, many people with dementia are vulnerable to disempowerment, through decisions being made for them, and may thus no longer be regarded as autonomous individuals, capable of making decisions for themselves (Parker and Penhale 1998).

4. *Creating purpose(lessness)*. In this fourth function of contested territories, the dynamic is used to frame purpose (and purposelessness) in the life of the person with dementia. In one example, Sarah seeks to mitigate her mother Margaret's difficulty in finding a purpose and activity in her life by emphasising her role as a grandparent.

In their study of social relationships when people with dementia are cared for at home by relatives, Askham *et al.* (2007) identify characteristics of Goffman's (1961) defining aspects of custodial care: routinisation, surveillance and mortification of the self. These characteristics were, however, all evident in the present study to varying extents and to various degrees are enforced and mitigated by the practices of the person with dementia, their family carer and their practitioner. Indeed, just as Goffman found, the people with dementia in this study used various tactics in an attempt to maintain their identity – drawing on our earlier case studies, Mary for example, sought opportunities to smoke (despite Peter's attempts of surveillance) and shared her experiences with friends. Walker *et al.* (2006) also identify that family carers of people with dementia adopt a role of supervision and worry that something harmful will happen if they leave their relative alone (however, unlike Bond *et al.* 2002, Walker *et al.* argue that the carers' judgement of the likelihood of harm is reasonable). Our research also supported the work of Mitchell and Glendinning (2007) who, in their research review, identified that risk-taking activities could be undertaken 'covertly' by older people without the knowledge of family and practitioners who were supporting them.

In everyday life there is a constant interplay between multiple perspectives, interpretations and their dynamic nature, despite there being regularity from routine and more fixed biographical dimension. It is in this dynamic nature of everyday life that the research we are describing illustrates how a person with dementia, their family carer(s) and practitioner(s) variously amplify and attenuate risk constructions, assessment and management. The importance of this is highlighted when considering the findings of Bond *et al.* (2002) who describe a diagnosis of dementia as possibly leading to professional judgements about lack of insight which lead to depersonalisation and loss of independence, these being irrespective of the probability of risk. In the Risk Study by Clarke *et al.* (2010), we can see that it is carers as well as practitioners who may amplify risk perceptions, and that practitioners are often seeking to attenuate the amplified risk perceptions of family carers and people with dementia. For example, Peter possibly amplifies the risks faced by Mary, and her practitioner attempts to mitigate this and attenuate the perceptions of risk. Similarly, Margaret's practitioner (like her daughter) seeks to attenuate Margaret's assessment of risk and encourages her to leave her home and engage in activities.

The purposeful dynamic of contested territories has implications for dementia care policy and practice. Risk assessments need to consider a wide range of perspectives, and in particular that of the person with dementia. Development work with practitioners, and family carers, can address the role they play in amplifying and attenuating risk. Contested territories can be explicitly assessed as mechanisms in which people with dementia make sense of their situation, maintain their sense of self and seek to continually negotiate their decision making.

It is in aspects of day-to-day life that living with dementia is experienced. However, aspects of everyday life become places, or territories, in which the place of dementia and the person with dementia are contested. We argue that these contested territories are purposeful, allowing for sense making, for maintenance of self, for claiming and relinquishing decision making, and for creating purpose(lessness) in peoples' lives. It is through these contested territories that the person with dementia, their family carer and their practitioner seek to moderate each others' perceptions of risk and explain and reconcile the changing family dynamics. Assessing and managing risk in a way that respects the dynamics and purposes of contested territories will support care that is person-centred, and moreover respectful of the relationships that contribute to maintaining the individual's sense of self and purpose.

SUMMARY

Fundamental to good risk management is the process of assessing for the views of all parties involved in the care of someone with dementia, and most important the person with dementia themselves. This chapter has described first some of the difficulties of achieving this, and the need, at times, to acknowledge and listen to the 'risk expertise' of people with dementia and their families because they are 'managing' the risks of the individual. Professional care workers are most likely to be orientated to the risk behaviours and actions of someone with a dementia and we will explore this in the following section of the book. In the latter part of the chapter, we illustrated the ways in which four people with dementia try to manage their lives on a day-to-day basis.

Chapter 3

Working with Dementia
Working with Risk

INTRODUCTION

This chapter will explore how risk is central to professional practice and how our professional lives are fraught with dilemmas that concern assessing and managing risk for and with people with dementia. To support this, we also outline some of the legislative framework in place to support practice.

RISK IN DEMENTIA CARE PRACTICE

Risk is central to professional practice, assessment and decision making and this is reflected in the growing emphasis on risk in UK policy (e.g. Department of Health 2007a). Titterton (2005) describes professionals as having 'to operate within a patchy and ill-defined context' (p.33) because theories of risk are often complex and challenging to translate into professional practice. Langan (1999) too, writes that 'mental health professionals commonly operate in conditions of uncertainty where risks are unclear and ethics dilemmas are rife' (p.154). As a result, practitioners can be reluctant to engage with risk in day-to-day practice and this prevents positive risk taking. However, the 'safety first approach' that dominates contemporary health and social care practice is problematic since:

- it ignores the other needs of vulnerable people
- it denies them the right to choice and self-determination
- it leads to a loss of a sense of self-esteem and respect
- it can lead to a form of institutionalisation with the loss of individuality, volition and an increase in dependence
- at its worst, it can lead to the abuse of vulnerable people.

(Titterton 2005, p.15)

The difficulty of a 'safety first' approach to dementia care is that its focus is on loss and challenging behaviour. It disempowers people with dementia and fails to identify the real meaning of risk for that individual. It is an approach that also fails to promote risk taking, yet risk taking is something that Titterton (2005) describes as:

> a way of enhancing people's lives; recognising the importance of psychological and emotional needs, as well as physical needs; promoting choice and autonomy for the individual; valuing the individual, irrespective of whether they live in community or institutional settings; promoting the rights of vulnerable people and their carers, while accepting that these will sometimes be in conflict. (Titterton 2005, p.16)

Hughes and Baldwin (2006) argue that the maintenance of safety can be replaced instead with a more positive 'ethic of care' which is characterised by:

- emphasising the importance of relationships;
- appreciating the uniqueness of individuals in unique situations; and
- a commitment to good quality communication.

(Hughes and Baldwin 2006, p.76)

Certainly, this approach to thinking about the tension between maintaining safety and maintaining autonomy is very helpful. Focusing on these more positive elements can help us avoid labelling people with dementia as problematic (being 'wanderers' or having 'challenging behaviour' for example) and allow us to support positive risk taking.

For practice, approaches to risk management in dementia care are particularly poorly developed and described, with many risk assessment tools being adapted from adult mental health services and the guidance on risk management in mental health (Department of Health 2007a) omits reference to dementia care. Indeed, where assessment frameworks are available, they tend to emphasise the importance of professional understanding with interventions geared to emphasise 'safety' and 'security'. The challenge for practice is to find ways of taking into account the positive aspects of relationships, individuality and communication when negotiating decisions in what can be quite difficult circumstances.

It seems that risk in dementia care needs to address cultural and societal expectations of mental health on the one hand, with expectations of ageing and older people on the other hand. In a major review of the literature, Mitchell and Glendinning (2007) found that in mental health the majority of studies concentrated on risk and 'danger' in which mental health service users were presented as a 'danger' to others or themselves. On the other hand, they found that studies concerning older people concentrated on everyday risks that older people encountered and the importance of risk taking for older people. In particular, Mitchell and Glendinning (2007) identified research which emphasised the need to manage risk in a way that achieved a goal of carers and people and dementia or disability to live their lives as much as usual as possible.

Think about – What do you think risk is about when working with someone with dementia or their carer? What words and actions do you associate with it? How does the idea of risk make you feel?

RISK DILEMMAS

In this section we have drawn on the survey we conducted as part of the Risk Study of service managers into the ethical dilemmas they were faced with in managing people living with dementia (Clarke *et al.* 2009). This can help us to think about some of the different ways that risk is understood in day-to-day practice and how that affects professional practice, as we discussed earlier in the chapter. The postal survey sample included people from health care, social care and voluntary sector organisations.

The managers described a complex system of interconnected decisions and actions with many stakeholders involved. As well as the person with dementia, these stakeholders involved professional and non-professionally qualified staff, along with a range of family carers, wider multi-disciplinary teams and organisations (themselves guided by frameworks such as health and safety legislation). One challenge is to disentangle these interrelationships, to understand which perspective comes from which stakeholder and how the one impacts on the other (how they reflexively influence each other).

A number of people in our research studies reported the importance of 'protecting' the person from possible harms of a physical nature. These included the possible consequences of wandering, driving and eating adequately among others. For example, an NHS dementia care coordinator described the following as areas of concern:

> People who may not be safe with gas, cooking appliances, heating – when to cut off gas supply etc. People who are reluctant to accept services but who may be eating or caring for themselves spasmodically – when to impose services.

Some felt that other people expected certain actions from them. One example given was being expected by family carers to lock people with dementia into their homes to avoid wandering behaviour. In such situations, the respondents are required to meet the needs of the person with dementia and in addition respond to the perceptions of risk of others (this most often leading to an expectation that risks are removed) (Titterton 2005).

As in any situation of seeking to meet a need, the resources at the disposal of the practitioner are an important part of their decision making. In this survey in the Risk Study there were two aspects of resource highlighted:

1. The resource of other members of a multi-disciplinary team who are able to work together to develop a shared understanding of the risks that the person with dementia is exposed to and can agree actions to modify those risks.

2. The care interventions that can be drawn on, and several respondents emphasised that a lack of service resource can result in undue exposure to possible harm through either under-responding or over-responding to a need. In under-responding, the person with dementia and their family remain in a situation that is judged to be potentially harmful with insufficient intervention to modify it. In over-responding, a higher level of intervention is used than is necessary, resulting, for example, in an unwanted admission to a care home.

Maintaining safety and protection from harm is, in the view of some respondents, insufficient. Many respondents advocated for the importance of proactive practice aimed at promoting activity in order to improve quality of life. The associated exposure to harm was regarded as a necessary part of achieving engagement, fulfilment and quality of life. For example, one practice development manager wrote that:

> Specific disabilities do create risks of involving people with dementia but we also feel that it is creating such opportunities with their inherent implications for quality of life that we should be facilitating.

These were at times presented as oppositions such as 'liberty versus sedation'. For example, one NHS service manager wrote that risk dilemmas arise from: 'Falls versus human rights; confidentiality versus carers' wishes; client wishes versus carers' standards; liberty versus sedation; immobilisation versus home support.'

The question then becomes 'which consequences are we as individuals (be it person with dementia, family carer or staff) and as a society more prepared to accept?' The lack of consistency in the consequences which people are prepared to accept, places practitioners and service managers in a very ambiguous position and means that we are more inclined to avoid threats of physical harm, even when so doing may compromise the quality of life of the person with dementia. Some respondents went as far as to suggest that the assumptions that underpin the practices of some service providers and some organisations are quite harmful to the people for whom they care. For example, the manager of one voluntary sector organisation wrote that:

> There is a tendency by purchasers to remove the person rather than the 'risks' involved. Clients are disempowered and their rights as citizens denied due to medicalising dementia and collusion of social services.

In day-to-day decision making situations, the dilemmas faced by many of the respondents concerned balancing independence and autonomy with exposure to potential harm. This balance requires reconciliation of two basic principles of ethics. The first is the universal duty of good clinical care – the use of expertise to protect the life and health of the people to an acceptable standard. The second is the universal duty to respect the autonomy of people. Clearly, these are the two issues that at times conflict with each other when caring for older people with mental health needs. Very often, the immediacy of the care situation presents multiple and sometimes conflicting avenues of action (Clarke and Gardner 2002). This is what Raines (2000) describes as an ethical dilemma: 'when two or more ethical principles apply in a situation that support mutually inconsistent courses of action' (p.30).

The dilemmas which people face result very often from the tension around the rights of people with dementia. In a study on continence management in dementia care (the Continence Study; Clarke and Gardener 2002), the ward staff were conscious of a duty of care to prevent harm to the patient (in this case, preventing skin breakdown in incontinent patients) but also felt they had a duty to respect the right to autonomous decision making of the individual. Furthermore, staff had to balance the rights of an individual with the rights of other patients in a ward as well as manage the sometimes differing expectations of relatives. They argue that, as a result, the ability to define, and deliver, good clinical care breaks down when 'good' continence care (as an outcome) is not always consistent with the need to nurture a trusting relationship with someone with dementia in order to provide 'good' care (as a process). As Hughes and Baldwin (2006) write: 'Judging what is best for a person is by no means easy!' (p.64). This is illustrated in the following quote by a practitioner who participated in one of our learning groups as part of the Risk Study:

> The carers will say 'Oh, they need day care, they need a befriender…they're not wanting it but that's what they need', and yet when you delve into what kind of person they've been they've always been a loner they've never wanted to mix… Again it's people thinking what's best for the person and going against what they're whole character and personality is.

Thus we can see that the dilemmas faced by practitioners and service managers in risk assessment in dementia care are indeed complex, and profoundly influence the nature of care available to people. The ways people respond to these dilemmas range from avoidance of physical harm through to managed risk taking to improve quality of life, and to an appreciation of the impact of organisational and professional patterns of behaviour resulting in harm to the person with dementia.

It is, therefore, essential that no-one working in dementia care should assume that their own perspective on risk is held by others and, not least, by the person with dementia and their carer. Obtaining information about the perspectives of others may help to illuminate some of the dilemmas experienced by staff in your own practice area.

Think about – As a team or an individual, think about the key resources which you can use or have developed in order to assess risk. In what ways do these resources allow for different perspectives of risk to be explored?

LEGISLATIVE FRAMEWORK

The UK law relating to mental health issues and to professional practice is complex and changes over time. It is not appropriate here to detail some of the specific laws and legislative frameworks – you need to ensure that you have up-to-date access to these and work within the arrangements put in place by your employer in relation to the law.

However, we do want to highlight three broad areas here. Carson and Bain (2008) provide a very useful summary, and we draw the following principles from their work. More detail is available from this resource too. There are three ways in which the law affects decision making, which we summarise here from Carson and Bain (2008):

1. When you are undertaking a risk assessment, the law may specify the *criteria* which must be taken into account. This happens, for example, when the Mental Health Act (England and Wales: Mental Health Act 2007) is enacted.

2. The law requires you to consider whose *values* are to be taken into account when assessing risk. In thinking about this, you need to be familiar with the Mental Capacity Act (England and Wales: Mental Capacity Act 2005). So long as someone is competent to make a specific decision and it would not involve committing a crime or endangering other people you are responsible for, then you cannot impose your values and your risk decision on another person. There are some people who are not entitled to make risk decisions for themselves, and this may include someone who has dementia. However, even in these situations, it is the specific decision that needs to be considered and someone with compromised or fluctuating capacity may be able to be supported to communicate and draw on their own values to inform a risk decision.

3. You also need to consider your own professional *responsibility* under the law of negligence. Under this area of law, so long as a professional makes decisions and acts in a way that is demonstrably consistent with what a responsible body of their colleagues would do, they will not be liable. In this way professional standards are upheld and reinforced by the law.

It is important, therefore, that these professional standards are clearly stated, perhaps in a risk management policy, so that the standards shape the values and criteria used when making a risk-related decision.

Understandably, people get very nervous about the *outcomes* of risk-related decisions – that someone may fall or get lost and so forth. However, it is really only possible to judge the quality of the decision-making *process*. A good process will, at times, and we hope very infrequently, still lead to harm being incurred. Perhaps more often, a 'silent harm' takes place though as a result of people avoiding taking risks. People with dementia are particularly vulnerable to what we can call silent harms – because staff try to keep people 'safe' by limiting the places they can walk in, for example, they incur the silent harm of disempowering them as individuals and making them feel helpless (or frustrated, angry, and leading to behaviours that challenge us). Carson and Bain (2008) write that:

> Quite simply, risk taking is sometimes a duty. Not taking a risk can be bad professional practice. Often the real problem is that too few, not too many, risks are taken. (p.36)

Think about – What are some of the silent harms that you see experienced by people with dementia? How much are your current risk-related decisions guided by what the outcome might be? Or by the process of making that decision?

BALANCING RISK ASSESSMENT

In this section, we will explore some issues about risk assessment that came from a series of collaborative learning sessions in the Risk Study with a group of around 20 people who work in dementia care and who were from a wide variety of professional backgrounds (e.g. social work, nursing, podiatry) (Clarke *et al.* 2011). These sessions focused on people's experiences of risk assessment and management in dementia care. There were three key interlinked issues.

First, the management of uncertainty by practitioners (and for many, the search to achieve certainty) leads to an interesting paradox. Working with a risk-adverse approach, prioritising certainty in which risk is minimised or removed, may nurture a level of competency akin to compliance in the person with dementia. It is a level that is adequate within the confines of a predominately '9 to 5' service. However, it may not best enable a person with dementia to manage uncertainty outside of times of service provision or uncertainty where a more 'expert' level of functioning is required for personal safety. Thus a focus on creating certainty, rather than the skills to manage uncertainty, paradoxically places the person with dementia in a position of escalating risk, being deskilled and increasingly dependent on service provision.

Think about – How are people with dementia deskilled by the services you know about? Does this keep them safe or make them even more at risk?

Second, amid complexity, professionals sought to weave a legal, physically safe and person-centred path through uncertain territory where certainty was most often privileged. Achieving this requires recognition of what was 'normal' for the person with dementia. Balancing the wellbeing of the individual and their family carer can be difficult and the focus of care could shift towards the carer. Decisions about risk management concerning the person with dementia are also influenced by the differing attitude towards risk taking of the professionals, their colleagues and of family members. In this way, the more people involved in someone's care, the greater and more diverse the perspectives on risk which need to be accommodated. Paradoxically, the more diverse the risk perspectives the more 'silenced' become the views of the person with dementia. To mitigate this, it is crucial that services and professionals consider who 'owns' the risk and is responsible for its management.

Think about – How many people are involved in the care of someone with dementia you know? How is the individual supported to ensure that their voice is heard? When a risk is identified, whose risk is it?

Third, professionals required special awareness or skill to understand and meet the needs of someone with dementia. We found that the mechanisms for gathering information about physical risk were comprehensive, but less established were the means for gathering information about the person and their psychological needs. Not only must comprehensive assessment be completed, including life story work, but this information must be communicated effectively to all staff and family involved with the person with dementia. Previous information gathered can be lost from present day information or overlooked by colleagues who privilege physical rather than emotional needs. Professional development needs to focus then not only on the acquisition of information, but its interpretation in a way that could repair risk and that balances the scales between physical and psychological risk. By risk repair, we mean the various ways in which people will correct or amend the outcome of an activity that may incur a harmful outcome. One example could be that of someone with diabetes who will 'repair' the potential harm of eating sweets by increasing the level of insulin they take.

Think about – Consider your present processes of collecting and storing information about individuals. How comprehensive is this assessment? How do you use this information to communicate with others and to make decisions about care? Are there key things missing or that could be improved?

The recommendations arising from our research (the Risk Study, see Appendix, p.114) focused on the following issues:

1. Attention should be given to ways of enabling people with dementia to manage uncertainty rather than create certainty since the latter may unwittingly lead to unnecessary dependence and risk avoidance.

2. Professional teams should consider how they collectively may be promoting risk-taking or risk-avoiding activity, and ensure that there is effective advocacy of the views of the person with dementia.

3. Professionals should review the comprehensive of their assessment, the extent to which physical risk is privileged (to the detriment sometimes of psychological and emotional wellbeing) and the ways in which information is communicated within and between services.

Let us explore the background to these issues in a little more detail through five issues that seemed to present contradictions or paradoxes, and each of which influence informing a balanced decision-making process. These issues were interwoven with each other and a risk-averse or risk-tolerant approach to managing risk in dementia care was also evident (see Clarke *et al.* 2011).

Seeking certainty

A clear institutional, family carer or professional's personal drive to achieve certainty in an uncertain world was apparent. Fear of injury to the person with dementia, which the practitioners thought could lead to legal action being taken or a complaint being made, underpinned a risk adverse approach to managing risk. This institutional drive promoted procedures and paperwork which were perceived as intending to serve the organisation:

> The risk assessment is the protective assessment of the organisation, if something is going to happen well it's ok if you've identified it, it's on the correct proforma, you've written down some...you're ok.

In practice, rules and guides can initiate the automatic thinking and recording of potential risks by staff rather than activating informed thought processes concerning the individual's needs:

> Well could I name them [risks], you don't think about it, you really don't, you just stick something down there and, and because somebody wanted you to write something.

A 'tick box' mentality towards risk management led staff to preconceived decision making about the individual's needs. Organisational legal requirements could dominate rather than a carefully considered review of individual need, shifting staff towards problem-orientated attitudes concerning risk:

> What she's [person with dementia] asked to do…are not great earth shattering things but they are being invested with all this risk around it.

Contrasting distinctly with a risk adverse-approach, were carers and professionals who prioritised individual needs, with a capability to reach the client in ways that are essential to expert practice and occurring only with deep involvement in the patient's situation. Balancing risks by maintaining perspective and accepting some degree of risk where possible was evident. This was also influenced by the individual professional's, family carer's or individual's personal approach to risk taking (e.g. a rock climbing professional empathising with the person with dementia wanting to pursue what cautious professionals might regard as risky activities). Some family carers and professionals accepted some degree of risk, with the professional team endeavouring to 'repair' risk while providing services, allowing the person with dementia more independence than otherwise possible:

> But we got a dementia support worker going in three times a day. And each time they were going in they were re-educating her. 'You know, don't put your tights on there [the fire]'.

Retaining some independence, this person with dementia learned to be safer when support workers were not present. Unlike the risk-averse approach, living with uncertainty was the norm for family carers and professionals who prioritised individual need.

Think about – Do your colleagues sometimes disagree about the extent and nature of risk for someone? Why? Do you have an assessment format that helps you to really think about the individual's needs? What factors help you make decisions that focus on the person with dementia?

Judgements

Linked to certainty was the need to make judgements to secure it, or alternatively to live with uncertainty. This includes making judgements and being judged, and some judgements were made for fear of being judged. Perceptions of being judged could be shared by both the institution and individual. Judgements were guided by several factors: an institutional risk adverse approach (combined with institutional or personal anxiety) and professionals' and carers' individual perceptions of risk. Individual perception of risk influenced respondents' comfort with balancing a fear of being judged with providing person-centred care. One respondent described how risk assessments frame the risk adverse approach to risk:

> The risk of the Trust getting sued, the risk of the organisation being sued in some way or shape…it remains a framework to be worked within.

But within that, staff make judgements influenced by workload and service availability balancing institutional requirements and individual patient need:

And if within that [framework] you look at risk, it's exactly like yourself, it's about the individual person but it's doubling the documentation, it's their judgements, it's hard.

Although individual people with dementia are the focus of risk management, professional decisions about this are influenced significantly by other family members. Professionals are also endeavouring to manage the expectations of family members and ensure that the needs of family carers are met, these not necessarily being consistent with the preferred approach to the person with dementia:

It's about the carers as well...really demanding on us to protect and make things safe. ...even though nursing staff are trying to work more towards personhood model, it's really hard for them I think.

He's got certain levels of risk and he's managing with support from services and he's in wellbeing but they're [the family] not happy to accept that. And it's a really difficult thing trying to talk to the family.

Acknowledging the personhood of the person with dementia is central to guiding professional judgements which focus on individual need. Institutional requirements, person-centred care and the individual's personhood were considered while attempting to bring some normalisation into dementia care.

Think about – What influences the judgements that you make about risk? What influence do other practitioners and family members have on your judgements?

Team working

The public and organisational culture is influential in the management of risk, nurturing either a risk-adverse or risk-tolerant approach. Where staff and carers were tolerant with risk, the focus was on the individual's own assessment of their need and creative solutions were sought to meet them. In the following example, and with the family also tolerant of risk, staff found a safe painting venue for this person:

> It would be very easy to focus in on those issues when you do your assessment 'Oh he's incontinent, better get the incontinence pads in' and maximise his personal care, and really what that man was saying was, 'I'm not interested in that, I want to be able to paint'.

Staff sought support from colleagues in making decisions about risk management but, as in the following quote, found this to be a fraught process at times:

> I sometimes don't feel I get [support] from…well particularly [health] colleagues. I seem to battle with them all of the time.

These findings highlight the importance of work cultures being supportive for person-centred care where risk is carefully considered and tolerated. Alternatively, risk-adverse approaches could initiate problem-orientated thinking:

> At times rather than deal with the actual problems that are in front of us we're more worried about the potential problems.

If couched within an illness culture which emphasises the deficits of people, options for creative solutions to needs are reduced. Furthermore, risk-adverse organisational and team cultures can be exaggerated by professionals' own risk-adverse attitudes. Where a strong risk-adverse culture existed, there is the potential for professionals to lose their 'voice' when advocating risk-tolerant strategies to colleagues, as described in the following quote:

I've sat numerous times in...case conferences sort of being the...championing the right of the individual and the carer against MDTs [multi-disciplinary teams] and it's almost to the point where I've actually said 'Well anyway if that's your decision, it's your decision, I'll record it as your decision' and you're thinking 'This is collaborative working?' You know!

Think about – Is your work environment risk tolerant or risk adverse? Has it ever been difficult to manage conflicting views? What are the strategies you use in order to negotiate different views to a point where you can take things forward?

Complexity

One further contradiction the participants experienced in their practice concerned the extent to which they were able to manage complexity. The assessment processes available to staff were at times considered insufficient to identify the breadth and depth of information the professionals were recognising as necessary to support positive risk management:

That's not assessment to me, that's ticky box. When I'm talking about assessment I'm talking about something more comprehensive.

Therein lies one of the dilemmas, you see if you want to be comprehensive it's often hard to avoid being lengthy and still being comprehensive. If you want to be brief you're not going to be comprehensive. I think that's a tension that's difficult to resolve.

The life stories of people with dementia were considered informative. In drawing a parallel with other services that require comprehensive and flexible responses (e.g. fostering and adoption), life story work was perceived to take relatively little time and so be a viable addition to the assessment of people with dementia.

The participants also recognised the time aspect of complexity. If assessment were conducted just once, it would fail to accommodate the progress of time and inevitable changes in circumstances. In managing complexity, 'trying to get a person-centred flavour into risk assessment' (practitioner) was paramount in enabling certain risks to be minimised. Typically, physical rather than psychological need was prioritised creating 'other' risks that may be deeply disturbing to the person with dementia, for example insisting on accompanying the person to the bathroom for safety reasons when the person with dementia regarded privacy as more important. Further complexity occurred when a carer's need, perhaps for respite, was inconsistent with the wishes of the person with dementia who may not wish to go to respite care. Both situations could create a decline in behaviour or health, creating another set of problems. Staff acknowledged that recognising physical risk was easier, not just because of its more visible manifestations but because its management and preventions was felt to be easier to address.

In addition to the tools used to gather information being sometimes insufficiently detailed for managing cases, the availability of services also influenced professionals' decisions, as in the following example:

> The problem of having a label of dementia is that we're now, sort of, perhaps pushing people into dual registered homes now, but they don't really need to be in dual registered homes, you know.

As a result, some staff were perceived to be reacting to potential problems rather than current ones. Conversely, a paradox could occur where a strong 'independent living' culture may be promoted but be inflexible in meeting individual need:

> I've got people living in the community who don't want to be in the community and because of the present policy of social services they can't go into care. ...because there

are psychological needs they would be better off in care. But that didn't even figure.

Think about – What assessment tools do you use at present? Do they enable you to describe the individual and their life in sufficient depth? In what ways would you change or improve them?

Gathering and using information

This study suggests there are two linked purposes of gathering information: identifying need for appropriate service delivery, and to identify and minimise risk. Emerging from the data were two strands of thinking: how best to *gather* information and how to *interpret* information.

Complexity could begin early in the referral process, with services being unclear about who required information:

> They're a Nimby, not in my back yard, it's a social care problem... We'll bung it to...social services or vice versa you know... It's a health problem, his behaviours are health problems, so we'll bung him back to health... poor person in the middle like a service user. (the Risk Study)

The inadequacy of information was emphasised, partly though limited assessment and in part though restrictions on sharing information due to confidentiality (especially between services):

> Partly because of time or, or whatever, you end up sometimes I think very, very often sort of with nothing really in enough detail about how people do manage to get on with life basically.

Gathering accurate, detailed information, which identifies the nature of the risk problem, enables staff to build and work from an evidence base. In the following example, concern had been raised about the suitability of someone with dementia taking a dog for a walk, the participant feeling that this 'risk' was mitigated by the benefits of the pet for the individual:

> It's a purpose to the walking, it's like giving them a purpose to go out walking, round the grounds of this hospital, they've actually got a...rather than just 'let's go for a walk to exercise your legs' it's about purpose, it's not wandering anymore it's a meaningful activity in walking.

A repeated or systemic failure to evaluate could add to the difficulty in interpreting information leading to 'misinformation' or belief concerning actual and potential risks accumulating. This may include the need to ensure time is taken to appreciate the views of the individual (which will take some time and skill) and to communicate information between different members of a team, as described in the following quote:

> I don't see it with everybody but then there was people who you know people with dementia who are talking in metaphors... And you can see that one person knows, will take some time, and will know and feed that back and that means something but then that stops because that person doesn't think that they're doing anything particularly skilful so they don't share it with the other people. That would make a massive impact on that person's lifestyle.

The participants described the skills and interpersonal relationship necessary to achieve a depth of assessment information with someone with dementia, and the careful observations of the impact of preventing physical risk on psychological wellbeing.

Think about – What happens to assessment information that is gathered and recorded? How are assessments shared between organisations, if at all?

The findings that are presented above help us to see how a practitioner working to support a person with dementia is in the position of having to balance their own policy and practice drivers with an approach that will ensure the best outcome for the person with dementia and any carers. The National Dementia Strategy for England (Department of Health 2009) highlights the need for professionals to have better education and training and the ways of understanding and working with risk is a key area for this better training.

Alaszewski *et al.* (1998) found three distinct roles in risk management were adopted by practitioners (in this study, nurses), though these were often blurred within individual practices:

- risk as a hazard and the practitioner as a hazard manager, a model that was more often associated with working in the mental health field

- risk as potentially empowering and the practitioner as a risk facilitator, most often adopted in working with people with a learning disability

- risk as a dilemma and the practitioner as a dilemma negotiator, a model most often found when working with older people.

Think about – Do you most often work as a hazard manager, a risk facilitator or a dilemma negotiator? In what circumstances would you adopt a different approach?

A key problem in trying to improve professional practice is the lack of understanding around how to balance the complex issue of risk, how to best assess risk and then how to manage the risk situation in a way that has a good outcome for everyone involved. When living an everyday life, people are making and negotiating situations continuously where risk is part of the decision-making process. In most cases this is done without explicit thought or discussion focusing on 'risk'. However, for people with dementia, their changing abilities and the shifts in the perceptions of those around them, places an increasing emphasis on the element and amount of risk in any situation when making choices and decisions.

SUMMARY

This chapter has provided a brief introduction to what risk is, and to why it is important to understand risk as more than physical harm. We have included some material from practitioners and management about the kind of concerns that they have, and we have sought to provide a basic legislative framework to guide practice. Moreover, we have sought to indicate some of the diversity of lay beliefs about dementia and views from a variety of cultural backgrounds.

In this part of the book, entitled *Different Views on Risk* we have explored how different people can have different views about risk in dementia care. These different views arise from the different knowledge bases that people have – people with dementia and carers having a very personal and individual view which they use to support a changing notion of themselves and their relationship; practitioners on the other hand have a knowledge of dementia which is built on learning and experience. We then explored how people use their knowledges in everyday life, and how for people with dementia, everyday life is where they seek to make sense of their changing life, where they seek to maintain a sense of self, where they claim and relinquish decision making, and where they seek purpose in their lives. We called these the functions of contested territories of everyday life, a concept that arises from one of the research studies we have completed. We then explored the ways in which risk can help us to understand quality of life. Whether we understand risk as something that is problematic or as something that contributes to a quality of life, we need to also take into account the relationship between the self and society and in particular the issue of who assumes responsibility for the management of risk. Despite policy moves towards individuals having greater responsibility for their own care, the evidence base of practitioners is privileged and the role of people with dementia and carers as 'risk experts' based on their own knowledge bases is diminished. As a result, the quality of life of someone with dementia is shaped by several global and social dynamics around risk. In the following section we will explore some of the key issues in the process of risk assessment and risk management.

PART III
RISK AND YOUR PRACTICE

Chapter 4

Risk Management

INTRODUCTION

In this chapter, we will focus on risk assessment and risk management. We will draw on two sets of data to explore some of the complexities of risk assessment and management in dementia care.

It is important that we recognise the work that has been done to develop risk management in mental health, and so we will here detail the '16 best practice points for effective risk management' that have been produced by the National Mental Health Risk Management Programme (Department of Health 2007a). However, this relates primarily to managing violence, self-harm or suicide and self-neglect. Obviously, these may apply to people with dementia, but our argument is that risk management in dementia care requires a more inclusive approach that will aim to maintain the independence and autonomy of the person who has dementia.

Think about – As you read the 'Best practice points for effective risk management' (Department of Health 2007a) in the box on pp.80–81, consider how each point relates to people with dementia. How can you build on these points? What else should be taken into account? In what ways can you think about risk more positively in your practice?

Best practice points for effective risk management

(Department of Health 2007a, pp.5–6)

Introduction

1. Best practice involves making decisions based on knowledge of the research evidence, knowledge of the individual service user and their social context, knowledge of the service user's own experience, and clinical judgement.

Fundamentals

2. Positive risk management as a carefully constructed plan is a required competence for all mental health practitioners.

3. Risk management should be conducted in a spirit of collaboration and based on a relationship between the service user and their carers that is as trusting as possible.

4. Risk management must be built on a recognition of the service user's strengths and should emphasise recovery.

5. Risk management requires an organisational strategy as well as efforts by the individual practitioner.

Basic ideas in risk management

6. Risk management involved developing flexible strategies aimed at preventing any negative event from occurring or, if this is not possible, minimising the harm caused.

7. Risk management should take into account that risk can be both general and specific, and that good management can reduce and prevent harm.

8. Knowledge and understanding of mental health legislation is an important component of risk management.

9. The risk management plan should include a summary of all risks identified, formulations of the situations in which identified risks may occur, and actions to be taken by practitioners and the service user in response to crisis.

10. Where suitable tools are available, risk management should be based on assessment using the structured clinical judgement approach.

11. Risk assessment is integral to deciding on the most appropriate level of risk management and the right kind of intervention for the service user.

Working with service users and carers

12. All staff involved in risk management must be capable of demonstrating sensitivity and competence in relation to diversity in race, faith, age, gender, disability and sexual orientation.

13. Risk management must always be based on awareness of the capacity for the service user's risk level to change over time, and a recognition that each service user requires a consistent and individualised approach.

Individual practice and team working

14. Risk management plans should be developed by multi-disciplinary and multiagency teams operating in an open, democratic and transparent culture that embraces reflective practice.

15. All staff involved in risk management should receive relevant training, which should be updated at least every three years.

16. A risk management plan is only as good as the time and effort put into communicating its findings to others.

THE IMPORTANCE OF PROCESS

There are equally some very straightforward messages about the process of risk assessment and management as a central part of professional practice which need to be clearly stated.

Risk assessment means making judgements about the following points (Titterton 2005):

- the individual's capabilities and coping resources (be they social, material or personal)

- the gains for the individual's physical, psychological and emotional wellbeing

- possible disadvantages and harms

- the values placed on the outcomes

- the consequences for the individual of not going ahead with the risk activity.

(Titterton 2005, pp.83–84)

Titterton (2005) goes on to emphasise that good risk management is about a process of compromise and negotiation. It involves the following steps:

1. Consult and communicate.

2. Prepare a risk plan.

3. Ensure that everyone signs up to this plan.

4. Share information.

5. Monitor and review.

6. Support staff.

We can add to Titterton's steps by including the ideas of Morgan and Wetherell (2009). They argue that risk management can be 'disabling' and that to move to more 'enabling' risk assessment and management plans the following important principles need to be introduced:

- information efficiently communicated, through a more collaborative process

- a transparent 'need to know basis' established

- a sense of ownership of documentation, developed through the practical processes of consultation and testing of ideas

- eradication of duplication

- an awareness of realistic expectations openly acknowledged by all parties, that risks can be minimised or reduced but not eliminated

- a recognisable culture shift to a more open use of risk-assessment information for the purpose of meeting service user needs rather than just a way to find out what went wrong, and who made the mistakes.

(Morgan and Wetherell 2009, p.254)

They point too to the role of confidentiality as both a major feature of professional practice, but as also leading to some major communication failures which have led to unnecessary risk taking.

The *process* of assessing and managing risk is important, as well as what it is that is being assessed (the person or situation for example). Titterton (2005) offers a useful simple model to guide the process – this is known as the Person-Centred Risk Assessment and Management system (PRAMS) and has five stages:

1. Staff discuss and establish 'risk' principles.

2. Risk policies are created.

3. Risk is assessed with staff discussing the appropriateness of different models of risk assessment.

4. Risk plans for service users and their families are devised.

5. Risk is managed, developing practical risk management strategies.

As you read on through this chapter, it may seem that we are trying to make things messy and complicated – introducing various different people's values and varying risk judgements. However, it is important to keep the principles above in mind and remember that risk assessment and management is about the *process* and how you engage with and document decision making.

RISK FRAMEWORK

The previous sections have illustrated how practitioners perceive risk and the concerns they face in managing risk, and then we considered how people with dementia describe their risks and the interrelationship between their perceptions and the concerns of their family and professional carers. It is useful now to draw this together to think about what might constitute elements of a framework of risk management. We can draw, too, on the work of Taylor (2006) in a study of social workers working with older people, who identified six risk paradigms:

1. identifying and meeting needs

2. minimising situational hazards

3. protecting the individual and others

4. balancing benefits and harms

5. accounting for resources and priorities

6. wariness of lurking conflicts.

(Taylor 2006, p.1417)

In a study of people with dementia living alone in Australia, Waugh (2009) found that professional staff addressed all of these paradigms as they sought to manage the 'competing tensions in providing person centred care in meeting the needs and addressing the risks of the older people who lived alone with dementia' (p.218). However, key to how risk was managed was the central importance of the relationship between the practitioner and the person with dementia. In seeking to make decisions which were in the best interests of the person with dementia in the face of complex and unstable situations, the professional staff drew on ethical practice and had to 'hold' competing tensions when, as often was the case, family, friends and neighbours were very anxious about the wellbeing of the person who lived alone and exerted pressure to move the person into 'safe' residential care.

A little work has been done to understand how relatives try to keep someone with dementia safe in the community. Walker *et al.* (2006) found that caregivers thought it was unsafe to leave the person with dementia alone, even when their dementia was mild. However, taking more safeguards did not reduce the number of incidents, nor did lower levels of incidents reduce the stress reported by caregivers. Risk-management behaviour was associated with both perceived risk and by the severity of the illness. The steps taken by carers addressed:

- *fire and/or water safety* e.g. supervision by carer, removal of items that could lead to fire or flooding (steps that we saw Peter take in relation to managing his partner's risks from smoking in Chapter 2)

- *caregiver taking responsibility* e.g. taking responsibility for finances (as we saw in Kath now managing Jack's finances)

- *preventing leaving the building* e.g. locking doors, hiding house keys

- *preventing falls* e.g. removing rugs, adding handrails

- *removal of dangerous objects* e.g. medication (or in Margaret's case, she herself stopped using kitchen equipment)

- *improving ease of checking on the person with dementia* e.g. moving closer to each other, phoning regularly

- *reminders* e.g. notices on walls

- *carer keeping a spare key to the house* of the person with dementia.

Buri and Dawson (2000) and Clarke (2000) identified how the relationship between carers and older people shaped the carers' approaches to managing risk and maintaining a 'normal' life. Management strategies were underpinned by longstanding relationships and identities of both the carers and the older people and by the wish to continue living together. As a result, sometimes an intervention offered by services (such as respite care) can be seen by a carer as incurring significant risk to their 'normal' relationship with the person with dementia.

In the Carer Study, Clarke (2000) found that carers used the following strategies to 'normalise' their everyday caregiving experiences and reduce the risks of physical and/or mental health to themselves and the person with dementia. These processes helped carers to balance their own needs, those of the person with dementia and the maintenance of a 'normal' life:

- *pacing*, in which carers restricted their physical and emotional contact to the person with dementia, and focused on the present rather than anticipating future events

- *confiding*, in which they 'off-loaded' feelings to others

- *rationalising*, in which they drew selectively on information provided by practitioners, accepting that which supported their normalising story but rejecting that which did not.

In a similar way, things that may seem inappropriate and challenging to us as practitioners may make a great deal of sense if it is possible for us to understand the behaviour from the point of view of the individual. Take as an example one lady who spent her day cutting up the clothes she was wearing – this caused great alarm to a temporary care worker until her son explained that his mother had spent her life working as a seamstress. Similarly, Pugh and Keady (2003) give the example of a man who wanted to sleep in his day clothes, it being one of the few things he could exert choice over in his life.

This is a very different way of framing risk assessment and management than that described in relation to most adult mental health care texts. For example, Norman and Ryrie (2009) identify the following risk categories: suicide, neglect, aggression and/or violence, risk associated with disability, physical and/or medical risks, self-harm, and others such as exploitation by others and abuse of others.

RISK COMMUNICATION

An essential part of risk assessment and management is that it is effectively communicated. This needs to be a set of information that is shared between and owned by a practitioner and the person with dementia (and their family where appropriate). Moreover, it is essential that there is effective communication between different agencies and practitioners if we are to ensure risks are not left unattended with a consequent heightened chance of harm to the person with dementia. In addition, through sharing risk information, opportunities for people to be supported to take life-enhancing risks can be maximised.

Sells and Shirley (2010) have developed a very clear and therefore effective way of communicating risk in a challenging behaviour service – they use a traffic light system to indicate:

- *Green* – Proactive (preventative: meeting ongoing needs), staff should be attending to the person's wellbeing (green for go).

- *Amber* – Reactive (responsive: identifies and addresses changes in behaviour and levels of distress), staff should be vigilant to a possible change in the person's mood (amber for be prepared).

- *Red* – Contingency (risk management: when proactive and reactive fail to meet needs), used when an untoward event happens and the care plan should be acted on immediately to maintain safety (red for stop).

(Sells and Shirley 2010 p.22)

There are three wider aspects of risk communication which need to be considered further. One is risk amplification, in which the harms from something can become heightened beyond a point which is necessary. This can sometimes lead to the second aspect of risk communication – that of moral panic, in which there is a disproportionate reaction from society. One example of risk amplification and moral panic is that of youths who congregate – which has led to newspapers referring to 'packs' of 'feral' youths and the clothing of a hooded top (or hoodie) becoming symbolic of incipient crime and intimidation. A similar process can affect people with dementia, with a growing social fear of a tidal-wave of older people with needs that exceed the capacity of a society to meet. There are frequent (mis)representations of dementia that escalate people's concerns – one example being the 'dementors' in the Harry Potter series of books (Rowling 1999), which suck the soul out of people and cause a sense of terror in anyone they are near.

A third aspect of risk communication concerns the timespan between someone behaving in a certain way and the outcomes of it. For example, the long-term health risks of smoking, which include some forms of dementia, can feel very remote to a younger person, yet the rewards from smoking are more immediate – it is so very easy to overlook the harm being caused. As a result some forms of communication seek to make these longer-term risks visible through social marketing.

RISK ASSESSMENT AND MANAGEMENT FRAMEWORK

The National Dementia Strategy in England (Department of Health 2009) addresses risk management, and in relation to this, recent guidance has been developed by Manthorpe and Moriarty (2010) which seeks to help ensure that good decisions are made about whether people with dementia are being empowered to take risks that may provide stimulation and excitement in their lives, while ensuring that they are safeguarded in a situation. They recognise that lowering or removing the risks of activities or arrangements that are important to people may reduce some risk but at the potential expense of their happiness and fulfillment. Removing risk may also affect any chances of re-enablement, such as regaining the ability to walk.

Manthorpe and Moriarty (2010) suggest that the following table may be useful to help assess risk because it allows a balanced approach in which risks and benefits are weighed up for particular activities. For example, this tool can be used when considering whether the person with dementia might go shopping alone (independence but might get lost), or continue cooking (enjoyment and preferred food but may have an accident). This scoring system helps to identify ways of reducing either the likelihood of something bad happening or the severity of the harm or danger. Using a score (1= low, 10=maximum, or high/medium/low) can be helpful in sharing and challenging ideas about the level of risk. To do this effectively though, you need to know the person quite well, or take the time to discuss this with them and their carers.

Table 4.1 Identifying risks and impacts

Risk area	What would be the impact if it happened?	Likely (H/M/L)	Severity (H/M/L)
Physical harm			
Emotional impact			
Loss of confidence			
Relationship changes			
Financial/ independence loss			
Overall assessment – overall judgement based on the H/M/L risks identified			

Source: Adapted from Manthorpe and Moriarty 2010, pp.50–51

People with dementia and their carers need to balance the risks being taken, ensuring that enough risk is taken to satisfy the person's wishes and needs, but that the risks are being managed in terms of safeguarding the person. It may be useful to be very explicit in identifying:

- How far does the activity contribute to the person's quality of life?

- What is the risk of harm to the individual of undertaking the activity?

This information can then be brought together in a 'personal risk portfolio' (Manthorpe and Moriarty 2010, see Figure 4.1) to allow a full assessment of someone's quality of life in balance with the risk of harm. Importantly, this immediately allows us to see the activity as the potential risk (and not the person!), and to think about how we can move activities from higher to lower risk of harm and have constructive discussions with the person with dementia and their families about how they would wish to do this.

Contribution to
quality of life

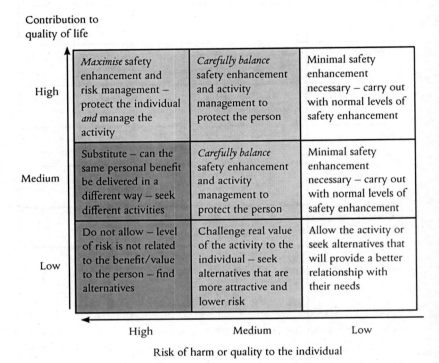

	High	Medium	Low
High	*Maximise* safety enhancement and risk management – protect the individual *and* manage the activity	*Carefully balance* safety enhancement and activity management to protect the person	Minimal safety enhancement necessary – carry out with normal levels of safety enhancement
Medium	Substitute – can the same personal benefit be delivered in a different way – seek different activities	*Carefully balance* safety enhancement and activity management to protect the person	Minimal safety enhancement necessary – carry out with normal levels of safety enhancement
Low	Do not allow – level of risk is not related to the benefit/value to the person – find alternatives	Challenge real value of the activity to the individual – seek alternatives that are more attractive and lower risk	Allow the activity or seek alternatives that will provide a better relationship with their needs

High   Medium   Low

Risk of harm or quality to the individual

Figure 4.1 Personal risk portfolio (Manthorpe and Moriarty 2010, p.52)

We would like to propose, therefore, that the following form a key framework for risk assessment and management for people with dementia.

First it is essential to identify what the risks are in the *life-context* of the personal biography and everyday life of the individual person with dementia. This can be achieved, for example, through life story work with the purpose of identifying the main factors influencing the way that the person wants to lead his or her life. This will include issues such as: physiological needs, safety needs, love and belonging needs, esteem and identity needs. It is this life-context that ensures that the person with dementia experiences purpose and satisfaction in life.

Second, identify risk *perspectives*, which include risk to the family and professional as well as the person with dementia. It is important to keep in mind that the individual, family members, practitioners, organisations and the general community (such as neighbours) will all have a different view of the situation. It is by being explicit in recognising these different perspectives that we can work out what really matters to the individual person who has dementia.

Third, the *weighting* of risks needs to be assessed (or think of this as the significance of risk). This needs to balance the advantages and the disadvantages of allowing or enabling something to happen. Remember how important it is to include the silent risks. This component of a risk framework involves attention to whether risks are being amplified, by the individual, by the family or by society, and awareness that this might be masking what the actual risk is. Weighing risks in the light of identifying different perspectives can help produce a well-informed and balanced judgement which is not distorted by the concern of other people.

Fourth, it is important to identify current and past *strategies* for managing risks. We can call this repairing risk exposure, and the person with dementia and family are likely to have already developed strategies for managing risks, so consider how these existing patterns can be built on to enhance risk management and provide safeguards. There may be an agreed plan of care to take into account (such as advanced directives). Identifying these strategies can help us work out the best ways of managing a situation and avoid proposing solutions that undermine and may harm the way in which people themselves are trying to cope and trying to maintain some purpose and satisfaction in their lives.

Think about – Read the introduction to this chapter again and consider how the emphasis there on process can be integrated into the above framework of *life-context, perspectives, weighting* and *strategy*.

SUMMARY

This chapter started by highlighting the importance of carefully considering the *process* of risk assessment, documenting decisions that are made and communicating effectively with other services, practitioners, carers and people with dementia. We then considered risk assessment and management from two perspectives: first, from the point of view of managers and practitioners, and second, from the point of view of people with dementia and their carers in their everyday lives. Finally we presented a possible risk framework in dementia care and highlighted the need for assessment and management to take account of the life-context of the individual, to identify different risk perspectives, to weight (or consider the significance of) risks, and to identify current and past strategies for managing risks.

Chapter 5

Developing Practice in Risk Management in Dementia Care

INTRODUCTION

In this chapter, we will revisit some of the key principles of the book and explore some of the wider issues concerning risk management in relation to quality of life, professional development and decision making. The management of risk for people with dementia will be explored in relation to the role of societal values, and the importance of having a focus on wellbeing and health promotion. In particular, this offers the opportunity to consider ways in which we might develop resilience for people with dementia, families and communities. We will conclude the chapter with a risk and dementia assessment framework for practice use.

REVISITING OUR KEY MESSAGES

In Chapter 1, we introduced a few principles or key messages of this book. We now expand on them here in order to consider the issues that have been discussed through the book.

1. *The 'problem' of dementia is not a problem which belongs to individuals, and it is important to refocus away from people with dementia to allow us to understand their interrelationship with the wider community and its impact on them.* Some of the aspects of this that we have explored are:

   - Reflexive positioning in which people adapt to each other in a biographical and day-to-day choreography. Any 'problem' is one that is shared and responded to with others and may not be seen by everyone as a problem.

   - The possibility of a counter-narrative of hope in the face of assumed tragedy and the search for meaning through biographical reconstruction.

   - Neither model of risk as problematic or as contributing to quality of life accounts for the complex interplay between self and society.

2. *For a practitioner, risk is something that is ever-present and which shapes professional assessment and decision making. It is something that can make us apprehensive (we may feel we need to 'cover our backs') and uncertain about how we might support people to 'take risks'.* Some of the aspects of this that we have explored are:

   - The importance of addressing the quality of the process of decision making about risk management, and of communicating this effectively with people with dementia, families, colleagues and other agencies.

   - There are significant dilemmas faced by managers and practitioners in relation to risk management, not least in seeking to balance safety and autonomy.

   - The law affects decision making in risk management in three broad ways: it can specify the assessment criteria to be taken into account; it enshrines the values to be taken into account when assessing risk; it addresses professional responsibility under the law of negligence (Carson and Bain 2008).

3. *Risk does not in itself mean something that is negative or harmful, although it is very often viewed in this way. Risk is a chance of something – this may have harmful consequences but it may alternatively have positive consequences which may enhance quality of life.* Some of the aspects of this that we have explored are:

- The definition of risk by Douglas (1990) as we have seen is a usefully balanced one: 'the probability of an event occurring combined with the magnitude of losses or gains that would be entailed.'

- There is frequently a focus on physical risk, but it may be more helpful to think of the tension between maintaining safety and maintaining autonomy and to recognise that risk is culturally specific.

- Risk as a concept and frame of practice is less well established in some countries, particularly developing countries, but its effects on people with dementia are none-the-less significant.

4. *Removing risk totally from someone's life is not possible or desirable because it would compromise quality of life, but it can be managed to ensure that harmful consequences are minimised and positive consequences are maximised.* Some of the aspects of this that we have explored are:

- The need to be aware of 'silent harms' for people with dementia, which can result from people trying to avoid taking a risk.

- The purposes of contested territories of everyday life are sense-making, maintaining self, claiming and relinquishing decision making, and creating purpose(lessness).

- Safeguards and risk repair help to support people leading their lives by mitigating some harmful consequences of risk taking.

5. *Different people will view something in different ways leading to multiple perspectives on risk. In such circumstances, it is essential*

that the person with dementia is supported to express his or her own perspective and the person's choices are enabled where possible. Some of the aspects of this that we have explored are:

- There are variations between the professional knowledge held by practitioners and the lay personal knowledge held by carers and people with dementia and which result in different values and perspectives of risk.

- Risk assessment needs to ensure that there is effective advocacy regarding the views of the person with dementia.

- Risk assessment must be comprehensive, to include everyone's perspective and be followed by collective decision making. As such, risk management is a process of negotiation.

RISK IN PROMOTING QUALITY OF LIFE

Risk mediates quality of life through a balance of risk taking and risk avoiding, there being an optimal level of risk exposure to maintain quality of life. This makes it very clear that avoiding all risk reduces quality of life and in so doing causes other risks – there is no such thing as 'risk free'. Together with many collaborators, we have been part of a research network on risk and ageing populations, and through this have developed a model of risk in ageing which will help us draw together the various threads that have been discussed in this book (Clarke *et al.* 2006).

We developed the terms 'risk-phobic' and 'risk-philic' to describe the continuum of beliefs and behaviours that seek to avoid taking risks and those that seek to promote risk taking (see Figure 5.1). Risk taking and avoiding involved:

- values – emanating from society and from an individual's biography

- choice making

- decision taking

- agency – of the individual and others to exercise their wishes

- negotiation

- risk repair – to compensate for exposure to risks that would otherwise result in harm

- safeguards – the protective processes that negate some of the consequences of more extreme risk-philic or risk-phobic actions.

This continuum is located within a series of concentric circles which represent different layers of influence and authority, each circle representing the individual, the family, the community, services, and the state. The interrelationships of the circles are culturally specific and dependent on each having the capacity for their own agency. For example, in India the notion of individual agency that is customary to people living in Western and more developed countries is not socially embedded and the agency of the family is considerably stronger. The ability of individuals to exercise their choices requires cooperation from others, or may be limited by others. For example, state authority in the UK denies individual choice over whether to smoke in public buildings.

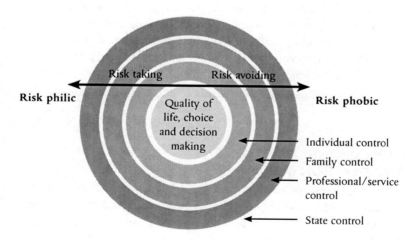

Figure 5.1 A developing model of risk for older people (Clarke et al. 2006)

In relation to risk and dementia care, we can identify how these different levels of control influence people's experiences. For example, in the UK, state control is arguably embodied in the Mental Health Act and enforced detention for treatment, and there is professional and service level control in both explicit ways (perhaps as the bodies who implement the law) and implicit ways (the resources available to them shaping the services and support available). In the earlier section about the contested territories of everyday life, we saw how the tensions between individual control and family control played out. Under the current personalisation agenda in the UK (Department of Health 2007b) we are seeing a move towards increasing individual control and although this is not fully developed in dementia care yet, it promises to give some choices and decision making (and the means to have agency to makes these decisions) back to individuals and families so that they are less dependent on professional and organisational determination of what services exist.

Think about – Can you identify the different levels of individual, family, professional/organisational and state control for people you work with? How can you increase the level of influence held by people with dementia? Do you have influence and control that has been given to you by the state, or by families and people with dementia?

PROFESSIONAL DEVELOPMENT AND DECISION MAKING

In seeking to reshape thinking and actions of any policy and practice, it is essential to consider how that professional development might take place. This is of particular importance given the emphasis on staff development in the National Dementia Strategy for England (Department of Health 2009).

In risk assessment and management, it is essential that professional development takes place in a collegiate way. Indeed, we discussed earlier how any individual practitioner's scope of action is shaped by the other people we work with. This will support us to do more than solve problems that build on existing assumptions (problem solving) and will help us and our colleagues to identify and analyse problems (problem setting). Eby (2000) describes this as critical reflection which requires self-awareness, reflection and critical thinking. Development that supports critical practice is essential – it has three components, each with an associated set of actions and skills:

1. critical action

   - sound skills base, used with awareness of context

   - operating to challenge structural disadvantage

   - working with difference towards empowerment

2. critical reflexivity

   - engaged self

   - negotiated understanding and intervention

   - questioning personal assumptions and values

3. critical analysis

   - evaluation of knowledge, theories, policies and practices

   - recognition of multiple perspectives

   - different levels of analysis

   - ongoing enquiry.

There are various ways in which you can engage in professional learning to support your practice developments. These can include: high challenge with high support, critical companionship, clinical supervision, Socratic dialogue, action learning and collaborative learning groups (see Clarke and Wilson 2008). Crucially though, we have already highlighted how important it is for the specific context of practice and of peoples' lives to be taken into account in making decisions. This makes a practitioner working on the ground with people with dementia, the person who is absolutely key to developing practice.

As one example, in the Risk Study we established a collaborative learning group with around 20 practitioners, meeting together for five half-days over nine months, with the purpose of exploring risk in dementia care. Collaborative learning groups combine the learning aspects of action learning sets with the research method of focus group interviews. Participants found the groups themselves to be a source of support and development: 'I think that what I have actually found from this group is just the support in risk taking, which I sometimes don't feel I get from…colleagues.' Participants described now viewing risk as something that could help them achieve more person-centred care.

> Prior to coming here (collaborative learning group) I would have thought risk, negative, litigation, let's just get rid of all risk. Well now I'm not, I'm thinking other people need to have that kind of perspective as well. So a tool (framework) that makes us all think that way.

Action learning has considerable emancipatory potential, especially if participants direct the issues rather than the facilitator or the organisation. The intervention strategies learned during action learning enable participants to increase their personal confidence resulting in them testing the boundaries of their practice. The learning potential of this approach is enhanced if participation is voluntary and learning is explorative rather than prescriptive.

Think about – In what ways are you supported to develop your practice at the moment? What suggestions can you make to your colleagues to increase the amount of shared learning that you have together? Are there different levels, from very short simple conversations, through to more complex change, that you can suggest?

Despite all of the emphasis on evidence-based practice, we know that in the day-to-day world of practice, the difficulties that practitioners are faced with are less likely to be about whether or not to implement research-based evidence, and are much more likely to be about what is right for an individual person with dementia and their carer in a specific situation. We can call this 'situated decision making'. Indeed, if research-based evidence were to dominate the process of legitimating practice then there are a number of undesirable consequences (Clarke and Gardner 2002):

- It stifles the creation of knowledge by practitioners.

- It compromises the accountability of practitioners to service users, imposing professionally defined evidence.

- It silences the knowledge base of the service user so that care may fail to build on self-management strategies.

- It fails to match the pace of change in practice so that practices often operate beyond a known evidence base.

Clinical decisions are a balance between the known 'best practice' and the expressed wishes of people with dementia and of their carers – and these may be different and not be easily reconciled with each other. It is essential that the value base of practice is clearly articulated so that there is a clear and shared understanding of 'best' practice. The situated knowledge of practitioners may result in optimal practice for a particular person in a particular set of circumstances (and this is quite different to the global nature of evidence-based practice). Martin (1999) also highlights how 'clinical judgements made by mental health nurses are time- and situation-dependent and consequently are unique' (p.273). Figure 5.2 illustrates how the different forms of knowledge need to be filtered through moral and ethical frameworks to create optimal practice through situated decision making. Absence of such moral and ethical frameworks, and failure to attend to the knowledge from evidence and from people with dementia, leads to situations of very poor care.

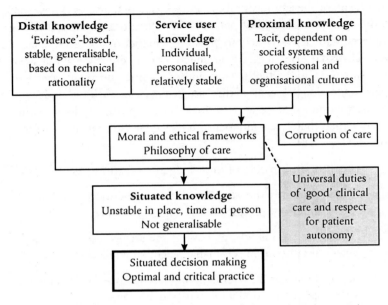

Figure 5.2 Situated knowledge and optimal practice (Clarke and Gardner 2002)

This again points to the need to have clearly stated values which practitioners use to inform decision making in risk assessment and management. Distal knowledge, generated by processes such as research-based evidence, is relatively stable and is important in underpinning defendable practice. However, the proximal knowledge of practitioners and that of people with dementia and carers, must be filtered through the philosophies of care and ethical frameworks that ensure that care is not corrupted by the values held by society. The product of these processes is situated knowledge, which is unstable in place, time and person. However, this does allow for the creativity and reflexivity of optimal and critical practice.

Think about – What are the situations of conflicting value and practice that you have highlighted to yourself as you have read this book? Does situated decision making help? How can you explore these ideas with colleagues?

CHANGING SOCIETY – MATTERS OF VALUE

In the previous section we highlighted that practice needs to be consistent with the values held by society. This is problematic though! Are practitioners to be led by these values, or do they have a role in shaping and developing these values? Of course, the answer is both. The values that society holds can be both helpful and damaging to the welfare of the individual within society, and this is crucially important when we think about risk in dementia care.

Minkler (1996) identified two paths of 'critical gerontology':

1. The political economy of ageing, in which the problem of ageing is located in social structures rather than with individual older people. This creates the structured oppression of older people by age being seen as problematic and by developing inappropriate definitions of need and care.

2. Humanism, in which the focus is on the meanings of people's lives. This approach challenges us to think about how society can support alternative and diverse definitions of age and ageing.

It is this second model of critical gerontology which the ideas in this book are seeking to promote – that risk management is all about people's lives in all their detail and diversity.

However, what we make of other people's lives is very complex – as is what we make of our own lives. Such is the stigma associated with ageing and with mental health, people with dementia themselves seek to hide their cognitive losses. The stigma exists because we have difficulty distinguishing between some ill-health problems and impairments and the sense of self and being. To be known to have a mental health problem, at least in Western cultures, is to bring the very essence of the self into question. The consequent destructive patterns of social interaction with people with dementia were referred to by Kitwood (1990) as 'malignant social psychology', and his efforts to highlight this and change practice radically reshaped dementia care during the 1990s. Kitwood and Bredin (1992) described four global sentient states which needed to be promoted if care is to be non-discriminatory for those with mental illness and those who are older. These states are an important today as they were then:

- a sense of personal worth

- a sense of agency (self-determination)

- social confidence

- hope.

There are many dimensions to the discrimination and reduction which underpin the care of people with dementia: mental health status, dependency, age, gender, culture, biography (denying peoples' past lives), the focus of care (onto the carer) and health status (ignoring some needs such as spiritual health) are just some. The many historical and cultural influences on the way that the needs of someone with dementia are understood reflect changes to the underlying social understanding of the role of cognition in society and in being a person. Reed, Stanley and Clarke (2004) make the distinction between self as a cognitive entity and self as a product of relationships. When the self is a cognitive entity, the effects of dementia are seen to be so pervasive that the person is substantially and irreversibly changed. They are socially diminished as a result and this allows others around them to distance themselves in order to define themselves as sane and normal. When the self is a product of relationships, people become increasingly reliant on others for a sense of self-identity. In a cognitively defined and dependent society, the society itself plays a part in disabling people with dementia. Reed *et al.* (2004) wrote that: 'it is the complexity of society that contributes to reducing the functional ability of people with memory problems' (p.81).

It is in reaction to these more damaging aspects of societal values and practices that people are now questioning the appropriateness of understanding dementia and dementia care in this way. Berrios (2000) wrote that 'the cognitive paradigm has become an obstacle, and a gradual re-expansion of the symptomatology of dementia is fortunately taking place' (p.10). We need, then, to focus on the enduring abilities that someone with dementia has, and not on their disabilities. And we need to be intolerant of places and people that cause unnecessary disability and social exclusion for people with dementia.

The importance of place of residence and socio-economic status cannot be under-estimated in particular as studies have demonstrated that the health of older people is perceived to be worse for those living in rural compared to urban areas. Indeed, the key factors identified by Parton and Green (2008) as influencing older peoples' quality of life were financial security (allowing independence and increasing health) and ageing in place and active involvement in civic or religious organisations. Cattan (2009) also emphasises the core sociological dimensions of gender, ethnicity, societal diversity, poverty, class and cultural differences which influence an older person's experiences of mental health wellbeing. In a multi-national study, Moyle *et al.* (2010) found that the UK participants, in particular, emphasised their experiences of feeling 'unwanted' in a society more youth-orientated. Given Sarkisian, Hays and Mangione's (2002) and Levy *et al.*'s (2002) findings that negative perceptions and expectations of ageing are associated with poorer functioning and increased mortality, it is clearly important to address societal attitudes such as ageism.

Think about – Think about people with dementia who you know. In what ways are they disabled and socially diminished by the people and/or environment around them? Can you share any examples of where people or the environment have prevented someone with dementia being disabled?

FUTURE DIRECTIONS

When we consider what the key features of a future for risk in dementia care could be, we need to acknowledge the macro-social shifts away (a little bit) from ill-health to wellbeing, and a more public health orientation to understanding the experiences of people with dementia. This creates the space to move from talking about risk, to starting to have a conversation about developing resilience. In this section, we will draw on two projects: a multi-national study into the wellbeing of older people (Reed 2008; Moyle *et al.* 2010) and a research network modelling health and wellbeing of older people.

The key to maintaining mental health wellbeing, as reported by a sample of older people (Moyle *et al.* 2010), seems to relate to older people keeping mentally active and their perceptions and participation in their community and relationships. There was little to indicate that older people seek to maintain and improve their mental health wellbeing through diet and exercise. Indeed, the association of cardiovascular risk factors, which are amenable to modification through health promotion activity, and vascular dementia were not acknowledged or discussed by the participants. This mirrors only in part the suggestion by Allen (2008) that wellbeing may be protected by taking an active grandparenting role, exercise, education and learning, volunteering, personal resilience, religion and respect. With the exception of exercise and personal resilience, all of these factors mentioned by Allen reflect aspects of participation in community and relationships.

In a recent workshop with about 40 older people (who did not necessarily have mental health needs), we asked the following questions (participants' answers are given too):

- What is wellbeing?

    o being an individual – through self expression ('having a say') and having control ('having control over my own life')

    o being valued – through dignity and equality ('not being classed as old')

- ○ a sense of peace and contentment – through peace of mind ('peace and balance'), fulfilment (being 'happy with myself') and contentment ('belonging')

- ○ having social contact – through company ('meeting people with a smile and getting one back')

- ○ having a purpose – through being busy ('motivation and drive')

- ○ feeling safe – emotionally and psychologically ('knowing you are loved') and financially ('knowing I owe nowt').

- • What would make it happen?

  - ○ finance – 'equal opportunities and access to financial support'

  - ○ cultural change – 'older people seen as a valued members of society not a drain'

  - ○ planning – 'don't make independent, dependent'.

Health care practitioners may be able to support people in their efforts to maintain and build community networks and relationships so that they can manage the transitions of ageing and family movement while encouraging the building of essential communication and network skills. Such an approach might be to encourage people to build communication and network skills so that they are enabled to connect and stay connected with society through, for example, telephone and computer communication, paying visits and attendance at social meetings. Such an approach will reduce the likelihood of people waiting for others to visit them and feeling disappointment if visits are not maintained. Furthermore government incentives may assist local communities to engage with others in their community through activities such as neighbourhood watch so that members develop a care and respect of people who are older or have mental health needs.

The findings have important implications for policy and health promotion. The exchange of ideas put forward by participants offers the opportunity to encourage an empowering environment for older people while recognising that older people themselves use several strategies to maintain mental health wellbeing. It is important that peoples' voices are heard by politicians and health care services so that policies and services meet the needs of older people, an approach advocated for also by Cattan (2009). Listening to older people through research will also help to determine what help is needed and how health care and policy makers can assist.

Given the number of strategies that older people use to maintain wellbeing these strategies need to be promoted within the community and linked to interventions that can be trialled to explore their role in assisting older people and in relieving burden on the health care system. Furthermore assessment and planning for maintenance of wellbeing for older people needs to take place in partnership with older people (Reed 2008).

Perhaps we are starting to see the effects of the Joseph Rowntree Foundation report of 2004 'From Welfare to Well-being'. In this, there is a reflection on the value placed on the individual and an acknowledgement of the aspirations older people have to retain independence, choice and control. It also emphasises that engaging more effectively with older people has been the most significant catalyst in changing policy. Page, Keady and Clarke (2007) write that

> We seem to be on the verge of a new and positive policy agenda which is influenced by quality of life, wellbeing, anti-ageism, social inclusion, empowerment and valuing the individual. It represents a seismic change that has led to debate about how best to commission, provide and deliver services, which not only reflect these ideas, but also identify and address barriers to change. (Page *et al.* 2007, p.17)

This is a mandate addressed too by the Association of Directors of Social Services and Local Government Association (ADSS and LGA 2003) who argue that the promotion of wellbeing needs to be given higher priority (see Figure 5.3). Most recently, the Institute for Public Policy Research (ippr) has undertaken a programme of analysis entitled 'The Politics of Ageing' (see for example Allen 2008).

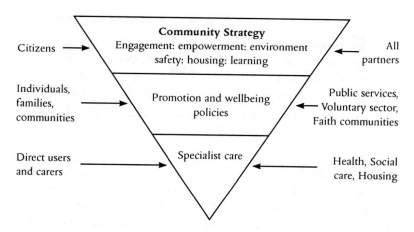

Figure 5.3 Support for people tomorrow (ADSS and LGA 2003)

It would be inappropriate to cast aside a focus on dementia as a disease process which has a profound influence on individuals and their families. However, this new orientation to wellbeing does open up the possibility of understanding dementia care in a positive, socially and community-centred way. It also offers the possibility of addressing not only risk but also resilience. Key questions for research and practice in the future include:

- What are the key factors which increase the resilience of people with dementia?

- How can the strengthening of resilience be built into risk assessment and management plans?

- What can families, communities and services do to increase the resilience of people?

- What steps are required of policy to enable this to happen?

Think about – How explicit in promoting wellbeing are you in your work with people with dementia? How could you increase or improve this? How can you identify what people are already doing to increase their resilience?

CONCLUSION

In this chapter, we have revisited some of the key principles of the book and explored some of the wider issues concerning risk management in relation to quality of life, professional development and decision making. We have also explored further the connection between managing risk for people with dementia and the role of societal values, and the opportunities presented through a focus on wellbeing and health promotion. In particular, this focus enables us to consider ways in which we might develop resilience for people with dementia, families and communities.

In this conclusion to the book, it is appropriate to reiterate a framework that we propose for risk assessment and management for people with dementia. It will enable practitioners to know of and build on the strengths of individuals and their families, and promotes a risk-aware care environment in which quality of life and wellbeing are paramount.

Risk and Dementia Assessment Framework

1. Identifying what the risks are in the *life-context* of the personal biography and everyday life. This can be achieved through life story work with the purpose of identifying the main factors influencing the way that the person wants to lead his or her life. This will include issues such as:

   - physiological needs
   - safety needs
   - love and belonging needs
   - esteem and identity needs

2. Identifying risk *perspectives*, which include risk to the family and professional as well as the person with dementia. Keep in mind that the individual, family members, practitioners, organisations and the general community (such as neighbours) will all have a different view of the situation.

3. *Weighting* of risks (or considering the significance of risk). This needs to balance the advantages and the disadvantages of allowing or enabling something to happen (and include the silent risks). Part of this component of a risk framework requires there to be attention to whether risks are being amplified, by the individual, by the family or by society, and awareness that this might be masking what the actual risk is.

4. Identifying current and past *strategies* for managing risks. We can call this repairing risk exposure and the person with dementia and family are likely to already have developed strategies for managing risks, so consider how these existing patterns can be built on to enhance risk management and provide safeguards.

Risk assessment and management are fundamental to professional practice. They can also fundamentally compromise or enhance the life experiences of someone with dementia and families. Attention to the detail of contested territories in the life of someone with dementia, to the history of people's lives, to the culture of societal values, and to the dilemmas and tensions inherent in variation between professional and lay perspectives and different practitioners will ensure a comprehensive risk assessment. Shared decision making and effective communication will contribute to achieving an effective balance between safety and autonomy. People with dementia can be among the most vulnerable and silenced members of our society – they also have enormous life experiences, capabilities and hopes. Effective risk assessment and management can help people to be fulfilled and confident members of their community and that is something we all have a role to play in achieving.

Appendix

This section of the book provides a little more detail about each of the research studies which we have undertaken and which underpin the ideas conveyed in this book.

FINDING MEANING IN CAREGIVING FOR PEOPLE WITH DEMENTIA (THE CARER STUDY)

Undertaken by C.L. Clarke as a doctoral study (1996, Northumbria University), the study aimed to provide a knowledge of the meanings of family caregiving for someone with dementia. It was a grounded theory study which involved a questionnaire survey of practitioners, interviews with 14 family carers who also kept a diary, and 9 case studies in which interview and diary data was collected from a different group of carers and all of their 25 professional carer contacts. The grounded theory analysis of constant comparison led to the development of a theory of normalisation.

Further reading

Clarke, C.L. (1995) 'Care of Elderly People Suffering from Dementia and their Co-Resident Informal Carers.' In B. Heyman (ed.) *Researching User Perspectives on Community Health Care.* London: Chapman & Hall.

Clarke, C.L. (1997) 'In Sickness and in Health: Remembering the Relationship in Family Caregiving for People with Dementia.' In M. Marshall (ed.) *The State of the Art in Dementia Care.* London: Centre for Policy on Ageing.

Clarke, C.L. (1999) 'Family caregiving for people with dementia: Some implications for policy and professional practice.' *Journal of Advanced Nursing 29*, 3, 712–720.

Clarke, C.L. (1999) 'Professional Practice with People with Dementia and their Family Carers: Help or Hindrance?' In T. Adams and C.L. Clarke (eds) *Dementia Care: Developing Partnerships in Practice.* London: Balliere Tindall.

Clarke, C.L. and Heyman, B. (1998) 'Risk Management for People with Dementia.' In B. Heyman (ed.) *Risk, Health and Healthcare: A Qualitative Approach*. London: Chapman & Hall.

Clarke, C. and Watson, D. (1991) 'Informal carers of the dementing elderly: A study of relationships.' *Nursing Practice 4*, 4, 17–21.

Clarke, C.L., Heyman, R., Pearson, P. and Watson, D.W. (1993) 'Formal carers: Attitudes to working with the dementing elderly and their informal carers.' *Health and Social Care 1*, 4, 227–238.

RISK CONSTRUCTION AND MANAGEMENT IN DEMENTIA CARE (THE RISK STUDY)

This study was funded by the Health Foundation in a grant held by C.L. Clarke, J. Keady and H. Wilkinson. C. Gibb also worked on this study along with A. Cook, A. Luce and L. Williams. The study aimed to understand the construction of risk in dementia care from the perspective of the person with dementia, family carers and practitioners with the intention of developing negotiated partnerships in risk management. The project involved a national postal survey of managers of dementia services, interviews with 55 people with dementia (frequently twice), and their nominated carer and practitioner, and collaborative learning groups with around 20 practitioners.

Further reading

Clarke, C., Luce, A., Gibb, C., Williams, L., *et al.* (2004) 'Contemporary risk management in dementia: An organisational survey of practices and inclusion of people with dementia.' *Signpost 9*, 1, 27–31.

Clarke, C.L., Gibb, C., Keady, J., Luce, A., *et al.* (2009) 'Risk management dilemmas in dementia care: An organisational survey in three UK countries.' *International Journal of Older People Nursing 4*, 89–96.

Clarke, C.L., Keady, J., Wilkinson, H., Gibb, C., *et al.* (2010) ,Dementia and risk: Contested territories of everyday life.' *Journal of Nursing and Healthcare in Chronic Illness 2*, 2, 102–112.

Clarke, C.L., Wilcockson, J., Gibb, C.E., Keady, J., Wilkinson, H. and Luce, A. (2011) 'Reframing risk management in dementia care through collaborative learning.' *Health and Social Care in the Community 19*, 23–32.

Keady, J., Clarke, C.L., Wilkinson, H., Gibb C., *et al.* (2009) 'Alcohol-related brain damage: Narrative storylines and risk constructions.' *Health, Risk and Society 11*, 4, 321–340.

CONTINENCE MANAGEMENT IN ACUTE DEMENTIA CARE ENVIRONMENTS (THE CONTINENCE STUDY)

This study was funded by an NHS Trust and was undertaken by C. Clarke and A. Gardner. This action research study aimed to develop an understanding of the challenges facing the development of continence care. Data was collected by focus group interview and non-participant observation. The study identified some of the ethical dilemmas faced by practitioners.

Further reading

Clarke, C. and Gardner, A. (2002) 'Dilemmas, Decisions and Continence Care for People with Dementia.' In S. Benson (ed) *Dementia Topics for the Millennium and Beyond.* London: Hawker Publications.

Clarke, C.L. and Gardner, A. (2002) 'Therapeutic and ethical practice: A participatory action research project in old age mental health.' *Practice Development in Healthcare 1,* 1, 39–53.

RISK CONSTRUCTION BY PEOPLE WITH DEMENTIA LIVING IN DISADVANTAGED COMMUNITIES IN SOUTH AFRICA (THE SOUTH AFRICAN STUDY)

This study was undertaken by C. Gibb as a post-doctoral fellowship. The study aimed to develop an understanding of risk construction and management in three different social groups of the Cape Town metropole in South Africa: black older people living in an informal settlement ('township'); mixed race ('coloured') older people accessing day and respite care in a poor community; white South African accessing a dementia support group. Data was collected by interview with people with dementia and a focus group with a non-governmental organisation in each of the three areas.

References

Alaszewski, A., Alaszewski, H., Manthorpe, J. and Ayer, S. (1998) *Assessing and Managing Risk in Nurse Education and Practice: Supporting Vulnerable People in the Community*. London: English National Board for Nursing, Midwifery and Health Visiting.

Allen, J. (2008) *Older People and Wellbeing*. London: Institute for Public Policy Research.

Alzheimer's Society (2007) *Dementia UK: The Full Report*. London: Alzheimer's Society.

Alzheimer's Society (2008) *Dementia – Out of the Shadows*. London: Alzheimer's Society.

Askham, J., Briggs, K., Norman, I. and Redfern, S. (2007) 'Care at home for people with dementia: As in a total institution?' *Ageing and Society 27*, 3–24.

Association of Director of Social Services and Local Government Association (ADSS and LGA) (2003) *All Our Tomorrows: Inverting the Triangle of Care*. London: ADSS and LGA.

Berrios, G. (2000) 'Dementia: Historical Overview.' In J. O'Brien, D. Ames and A. Burn (eds) *Dementia* (2nd edition). London: Arnold.

Bond, J., Corner, L., Lilley, A. and Ellwood, C. (2002) 'Medicalization of insight and caregivers' responses to risk in dementia.' *Dementia 1, 3*, 313–28.

Buri, H. and Dawson, P. (2000) 'Caring for a relative with dementia: A theoretical model of coping with fall risk.' *Health, Risk and Society 2*, 283–93.

Bury, M. (1991) 'The sociology of chronic illness: A review of research and prospects.' *Sociology of Health and Illness 13*, 4, 451–468.

Carson, D. and Bain, A. (2008) *Professional Risk and Working with People*. London: Jessica Kingsley Publishers.

Cattan, M. (ed.) (2009) *Mental Health and Well-Being in Later Life*. Maidenhead: Open University Press.

Clarke, C.L. (1997) 'In Sickness and in Health: Remembering the Relationship in Family Caregiving for People with Dementia.' In M. Marshall (ed.) *State of the Art in Dementia Care*. London: Centre for Policy on Ageing.

Clarke, C. (2000) 'Risk: Constructing care and care environments in dementia.' *Health, Risk and Society 2*, 83–93.

Clarke, C. and Gardner, A. (2002) 'Dilemmas, Decisions – and Continence Care for People with Dementia.' In S. Benson (ed.) *Dementia Topics for the Millennium and Beyond*. London: Hawker Publications.

Clarke, C.L. and Heyman, B. (1998) 'Risk Management for People with Dementia.' In B. Heyman (ed.) *Risk, Health and Health Care.* London: Arnold.

Clarke, C.L. and Keady, J. (1996) 'Researching dementia care and family caregivers: Extending ethical responsibilities.' *Health Care in Later Life 1,* 2, 85–95.

Clarke, C.L. and Wilson, V. (2008) 'Learning – The Heart of Practice Development.' In K. Manley, B. McCormack and V. Wilson (eds) *International Practice Development in Nursing and Healthcare.* Chichester: Blackwell Publishing.

Clarke, C.L. and members of the International Collaborative Research Network on Risk and Ageing Populations (2006) 'Risk and ageing populations: Development research through an international research network.' *International Journal of Older People Nursing 1,* 3, 169–176.

Clarke, C.L., Gibb, C., Keady, J., Luce, A., *et al.* (2009) 'Risk management dilemmas in dementia care: An organisational survey in three UK countries.' *International Journal of Older People Nursing 4,* 89–96.

Clarke, C.L., Keady, J., Wilkinson, H., Gibb, C., *et al.* (2010) 'Dementia and risk: Contested territories of everyday life.' *Journal of Nursing and Healthcare of Chronic Illness 2,* 102–112.

Clarke, C.L., Wilcockson, J., Gibb, C.E., Keady, J., Wilkinson, H. and Luce, A. (2011) Reframing risk management in dementia care through collaborative learning.' *Health and Social Care in the Community 19,* 23–32.

Crisp, J. (1999) 'Towards a Partnership in Maintaining Personhood.' In T. Adams and C.L. Clarke (eds) *Dementia Care: Developing Partnerships in Practice.* London: Bailliere Tindall.

Daker-White, G., Beattie, A., Means, R. and Gilleard, J. (2002) *Service the Needs of Marginalised Groups in Dementia Care: Younger People and Minority Ethnic Groups.* Bristol: University of the West of England and Dementia Voice.

Department of Health (2007a) *Best Practice in Managing Risk.* London: Department of Health.

Department of Health (2007b) *Putting People First: A Shared Vision and Commitment to the Transformation of Adult Social Care.* London: Department of Health.

Department of Health (2009) *Living Well with Dementia: A National Dementia Strategy.* London: Department of Health.

Douglas, M. (1990) 'Risk as a forensic resource.' *Daedalus, Journal of the American Academy of Arts and Science 119,* 1–16.

Douglas, M. (1994) *Risk and Blame: Essays in Cultural Theory.* London: Routledge.

Eby, M. (2000) 'Understanding Professional Development.' In A. Brechin, H. Brown and M.A. Eby (eds) *Critical Practice in Health and Social Care.* London: Sage.

England and Wales (2005) *Mental Health Act 2005 Elizabeth II.* London: The Stationery Office

England and Wales (2008) *Mental Health Act 2007 Elizabeth II.* London: The Stationery Office.

Ferreira, M. and Makoni, S.B. (1999) 'Towards a Cultural and Linguistic Construction of Late-life Dementia in an Urban African Population.' In S.B. Makoni and K. Stroeken (eds) *Ageing in Africa: Sociolinguistic and Anthropological Approaches.* Aldershot: Ashgate.

Fortinsky, R., Panzer, V. and Wakefield, F.I. (2009) 'Alignment between falls risk and balance confidence in later life: Has over-confidence been overlooked?' *Health, Risk and Society 11,* 4, 341–352.

Galvin, K., Todres, L. and Richardson, M. (2005) 'The intimate mediator: A carer's experience of Alzheimer's.' *Scandinavian Journal of Caring Sciences 19*, 2–11.

Gates, K. (2000). 'The experience of caring for a loved one: A phenomenological study.' *Nursing Science Quarterly 13*, 54–59.

Goffman, E. (1961) *Asylums: Essays on the Social Situation of Mental Patients and Other Inmates.* New York: Anchor.

Hughes, J.C. and Baldwin, C. (2006) *Ethical Issues in Dementia Care.* London: Jessica Kingsley. Publishers.

Illiffe, S. and Manthorpe, J. (2004) 'The hazards of early recognition of dementia: A risk assessment.' *Ageing and Mental Health 8*, 2, 99–105.

Joseph Rowntree Foundation (2004) *From Welfare to Well-Being – Planning for an Ageing Society: Summary Conclusions of the Joseph Rowntree Foundation Task Group on Housing, Money and Care for Older People.* Available at www.jrf.org.uk/sites/files/jrf/034.pdf, accessed on 18 January 2011.

Kalaria, R.N., Maestre, G.E., Arizaga, R., Friedland, R.P., *et al.* (2008) 'Alzheimer's disease and vascular dementia in developing countries: Prevalence, management, and risk factors.' *Lancet Neurology 7*, 9, 812–826.

Keady, J., Clarke, C.L., Wilkinson, H., Williams, L., *et al.* (2009) 'Alcohol-related brain damage: Narrative storylines and risk constructions.' *Health, Risk and Society 11*, 4, 321–340.

Kitwood, T. (1990) 'The dialectics of dementia: With particular reference to Alzheimer's disease.' *Ageing and Society 10*, 177–96.

Kitwood, T. (1997) *Dementia Reconsidered: The Person Comes First.* Maidenhead: Open University Press.

Kitwood, T. and Bredin, K. (1992) 'Towards a theory of dementia care: Personhood and wellbeing.' *Ageing and Society 12*, 269–87.

Langan, J. (1999) 'Assessing Risk in Mental Health.' In P. Parsloe (ed) *Risk Assessment in Social Care and Social Work.* London: Jessica Kingsley Publishers.

Levy, B.R., Slade, M.D., Kunkel, S.R. and Karsi, S.V. (2002) 'Longevity increased by positive self-perceptions of aging.' *Journal of Personality and Social Psychology 83*, 261–270.

Manthorpe, J. and Moriarty, J. (2010) *Nothing Ventured, Nothing Gained: Risk Guidance for People with Dementia.* London: Department of Health.

Martin, P.J. (1999) 'Influences on clinical judgement in mental health nursing.' *Nursing Times Research 4*, 273–280.

Minkler, M. (1996) 'Critical perspectives of ageing: New challenges for gerontology.' *Ageing and Society 16*, 467–487.

Mitchell, W. and Glendinning, C. (2007) *A Review of the Research Evidence Surrounding Risk Perceptions, Risk Management Strategies and their Consequences in Adult Social Care for Different Groups of Service Users.* York: University of York, Social Policy Research Unit.

Morgan, S. and Wetherell, A. (2009) 'Working with Risk.' In I. Norman and I. Ryrie (eds) *The Art and Science of Mental Health Nursing.* Maidenhead: Open University Press.

Moyle, W., Clarke, C.L., Gracia, N., Reed, J., et al. (2010) 'Older people maintaining mental health well-being through resilience: An appreciative inquiry study in four countries.' Journal of Nursing and Healthcare in Chronic Illness 2, 113–121.

National Institute for Health and Clinical Excellence (NICE) and the Social Care Institute for Excellence (SCIE) (2007) Dementia: Supporting People with Dementia and their Carers in Health and Social Care (NICE clinical practice guideline 42: NICE/SCIE 2006). Leicester: The British Psychological Society.

Nolan, M., Davies, S., Ryan, T. and Keady, J. (2008) 'Relationship-centred care and the "senses" framework.' Journal of Dementia Care 16, 1, 26–28.

Nuffield Council on Bioethics (2009) Dementia: Ethical Issues. London: Nuffield Council.

Oulton, K. and Heyman, B. (2009) 'Devoted protection: How parents of children with severe learning disabilities manage risks.' Health, Risk and Society 11, 4, 303–319.

Page, S., Keady, J. and Clarke, C.L. (2007) 'Models of Community Support for People with Dementia.' In J.Keady, C.L. Clarke and S. Page (eds) Partnerships in Community Mental Health Nursing and Dementia Care: Practice Perspectives. Maidenhead: Open University Press.

Parker, J. and Penhale, B. (1998) Forgotten People: Positive Approaches to Dementia Care. Aldershot: Ashgate.

Parton, S. and Green, S. (2008) 'A comparison of subjective quality-of-life indicators across domains of Jewish seniors living in the community.' Social Work / Maatskaplike 44, 2, 107–124.

Powell J., Wahidin A. and Zinn J. (2007) 'Understanding risk and old age in western society.' International Journal of Sociology and Social Policy 27, 65–76.

Prince, M., Graham, N., Brodaty, H., Rimmer, E., et al. (2004) 'Alzheimer Disease International's 10/66 Dementia Research Group – One model for action research in developing countries.' International Journal of Geriatric Psychiatry 19, 2, 178–181.

Pugh, M. and Keady, J. (2003) 'Assessing and responding to challenging behaviour in dementia: A focus for community mental health nursing practice.' In J., Keady , C. Clarke and T. Adams (eds) Community Mental Health Nursing and Dementia Care: Practice Perspectives. Buckingham: Open University Press.

Raines, M.L. (2000) 'Ethical decision making in nurses: Relationships among moral reasoning, coping style, and ethical stress.' Journal of Nursing Administration (Healthcare Law, Ethics, and Regulation) 2, 1, 29–41.

Reed, J. (2008) 'Older people maintaining well-being: Implications for future development.' International Journal of Older People Nursing 3, 76–77.

Reed, J., Stanley, D. and Clarke, C. (2004) Health, Well-being and Older People. Bristol: Policy Press.

Republic of South Africa (RSA) (2006) Older Persons Act No. 13 of 2006. Government Gazette 497 (29346). Cape Town. 2 November 2006. Pretoria: Government Printers.

Rowling, J.K. (1999) Harry Potter and the Prisoner of Azkaban. New York: Scholastic.

Sarkisian, C.A., Hays, R.D. and Mangione, C.M. (2002) 'Do older people expect to age successfully? The association between expectations regarding ageing and beliefs regarding healthcare seeking among older people.' The Journal of American Geriatrics Society 50, 11, 1837–1843.

Sells, D. and Shirley, L. (2010) 'Person-centred risk management: The Traffic Light approach.' *Journal of Dementia Care 18*, 5, 21–23.

Swain, J., French, S. and Cameron, C. (2003) *Controversial Issues in a Disabling Society.* Maidenhead: Open University Press.

Taylor, B. (2006) 'Risk management paradigms in health and social care services for professional decision making on the long-term care of older people.' *British Journal of Social Work 36*, 1411–1429.

Titterton, M. (2005) *Risk and Risk-Taking in Health and Social Care.* London: Jessica Kingsley Publishers.

Todres, L. and Galvin, K. (2006) 'Caring for a partner with Alzheimer's disease: Intimacy, loss and the life that is possible.' *International Journal of Qualitative Studies on Health and Well-Being 1*, 1, 50–61.

United Nations (2007) *World Population Ageing 2007.* New York: United Nations, Department of Economic and Social Affairs. Available at http://www.un.org/esa/population/publications/ageing/Graph.pdf, accessed on 5 April 2006.

Walker, A.E., Livingston, G., Cooper, C.A., Katona, C.L.E. and Kitchen, G.L. (2006) 'Caregivers' experience of risk in dementia: The LASER-AD Study.' *Ageing and Mental Health 10*, 5, 532–538.

Waugh, F. (2009) 'Where does risk feature in community care practice with older people with dementia who live alone?' *Dementia 8*, 2, 205–222.

Subject Index

Author Index